THE **IVDD HANDBOOK**

Helping your dog through back and neck problems

———————

DR MARIANNE DORN
'The Rehab Vet'

The IVDD Handbook

Updated November 2022

© Marianne Dorn 2022

ISBN: 979-8-351305-09-7

Cover photographs, clockwise from top left:
Burt owned by Vicky Watt-Hedges, Walter owned by Rachel Williams, Ernie owned by Elaine Brechin and Kenny owned by Abbie.

Hand-drawn illustrations by Marianne Dorn
Designed by Justine Elliott of Design Lasso

This book is written in British English.

Disclaimer
This book provides home care guidelines and includes background information to help you make decisions on behalf of your dog when your vet asks you to do so. However, it is not a substitute for medical advice and should be used only in conjunction with talking to your own vet. The author is not liable for any damages or negative consequences that may result from using this book.

Acknowledgements

This book is dedicated to all dogs who have been through, or are yet to experience, back or neck problems. Whatever your stage of recovery, I wish you strength and comfort.

I aimed to create a practical home reference for dog owners to turn to at each stage of recovery. This could not have been achieved without the help of many other people. Special thanks go to my husband, Alan, who tirelessly checked each stage of the manuscript. And a big thank you to my daughter, Ella, who advised on making the text accessible for dog owners. I am also grateful to Justine of Design Lasso for her patience and skill in making this book attractive to readers.

Many thanks to the following professionals for taking the time to read and comment on sections of my manuscript: Professor Paul Freeman (European & RCVS Specialist in Veterinary Neurology), Dr Andria Cauvin (European & RCVS Specialist in Veterinary Internal Medicine – Companion Animals), Caroline Clark (ABTC Registered Clinical Animal Behaviourist and Registered Veterinary Nurse), Vicky Burrell (RSPCA Branch Operations Manager) and Dr Heike Kopac-Pickering (president of ABVA). I am also very grateful for information supplied by Claire Defries (Registered Veterinary Nurse) and Dr Laura Hamilton BVM&S PgC(SAC) MRCVS (Kennel Club breed health coordinator for French bulldogs).

Special thanks to Ian Seath BSc (Hons) for his guidance and for writing the foreword. I would also like to thank the following dog owners and canine professionals who gave advice, encouragement and practical support at every stage of the book's creation: Julie Austin, Charlotte Baldwin, Elaine Brechin, Vanessa Bryant, Camila Castro, Maia D'Costa-Kalsi, Kathleen Gregory, Gill Key, Vivienne Kosviner, Vicky Watt-Hedges, Tim and Lisa West and Rachel Williams.

Finally, I am particularly grateful to one of my teachers, Barbara Houlding, for inspiring me to share information with others, and for reminding me to see each situation both from the dog's and from the owner's point of view.

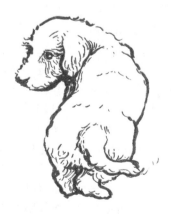

Picture credits

A huge thank you to the many dog owners and carers who supplied photos for use in this book. Your pictures of these lovely dogs will lift readers' spirits and help show what is possible during recovery.

Key: t = top; b = bottom; m = middle; l = left; r = right

Alfie owned by Rachael Power: 128bl, 191t & br; **Arthur** owned by Katie Field: 122r; **Attie** owned by Maia D'Costa-Kalsi and family: back cover tr, 17r, 36, 43r, 46tl & tr, 54, 67br, 68, 69t, 70bl, 80t, 84, 85t, 91t, 98b, 105m, 111, 112b, 113b, 116, 117b, 120t, 137, 142b, 143-147, 149l, 151t, 166t, 173, 176m, 183t, 188b; **Baxter** owned by Bernadette Pegorsch: 184b, 185tr; **Bean** owned by Christian and Lena 46b, 86t, 86b, 139m, 142t, 168bl, 169; **Bella** owned by Julie Austin: back cover tl, 38l, 43bl, 98t, 98m, 176t, 181tr, 212b, 216m; **Bella** owned by Sally Winup: 39, 64t, 187b, 188m; **Benji** owned by Claire Ellis: 45b, 60t; **Bertie** owned by Shirley 129; **Billy** owned by Luke and Claire Cain 88tl; **Bonnie** owned by Abbie: 95b; **Buddy** owned by Bernie Bowling: 94; **Burt** owned by Vicky Watt-Hedges: front cover tl, 21b, 44, 45t, 47, 53, 79t, 86m, 117t, 133tr, 151b; **Catcher** owned by Anna Richardson 182t, 186b, 241t; **Cleo** owned by Irene Ferdinand: 81, 83b; **Cocoa** owned by Susan Riddle: 14r, 17l, 34; **Cookie** owned by Melanie Bruder: 71, 73; **Dappy:** 102l, 108, 138m, 187m, 234; **Darcy Dolittle** owned by Tim and Lisa West: back cover bl, 21ml & mr, 38r, 42t, 48t, 65b, 67bl, 74b, 76, 77, 79m, 87tr, 90b, 95t, 96, 99m, 100m, 102r, 103t, 107, 109b, 115b, 119, 133tl, 156, 170, 171b, 172b, 174tr & m, 175t, 176b, 177, 178b, 179, 181tl, 183b, 184m, 198b, 215b; **Digby** owned by Charlie Nelson: 203t, 204t & m, 205t; **Dillon** owned by Luke and Claire Cain: 88tr, 88b; **Elsie** owned by Rosy Pigott: 27m, 138b; **Ernie** owned by Elaine Brechin: front cover br, 19r, 32b, 52t, 112t, 128r, 134, 191r & l, 192t & b; **Feargal** owned by Terrie Ellis: 32t, 41b, 43t, 90t, 103b, 110, 127b; **Finley:** 61l, 70tr, 215t; **Frankie** owned by Helen Gouldstone 40, 58r, 135, 138tl, 139b; **Freddy** owned by Diana Krcmar: 72, 184t; **George** owned by Jenny Barrett 112m; **Goliath** owned by Paula Sayer: 19l; **Gracie** owned by Mrs Patricia Endersby: 97m; **Harvey** owned by Gillian Hamilton: 18tl & br, 35t, 188t; **Hector** owned by Lindsay O'Dell: 21t, 78, 83t; **Hector** owned by Ali Robinson: 64b, 216b; **Helen** owned by Mrs Patricia Endersby: 97t; **Holly** owned by Mandy Walker 162m & b; **Iris** owned by Nicky Loveless: 67t; **Kenny** owned by Abbie (with special thanks to Jemma for helping): front cover bl, 136, 147b, 148, 165b, 166b, 206, 208; **Louis** owned by the Hurford family: 59b; **Minnie** owned by Sarah Burton: 20; **Nate** owned by Vanessa Bryant: 83m, 105b, 163, 164, 172t, 175b; **Pebble** owned by Patricia May: 55b; **Princess Frankie Moore** owned by Nina Moore of Black & Tan Dachshund Boarding: 80m; **Puppy** owned by Camila Castro: 155, 157b; **Ragnar** owned by Dr Zoe Judd: 22; **Rio** owned by Vanessa Bryant: 133bl, 165t, 167b, 168t; **Roxy** owned by Tessa Lewis: 204b; **Rupert** owned by The Merrin Family: 66; **Saffy** owned by Julie Austin: 74t, 87b, 90m, 160, 161, 239, 241bl; **Taz** owned by Kate Daubney: 63, 70tl; **Teddy** owned by Sophia Agiadis: 123t; **Tess** owned by Jan Wrench and Nathan Hughes: 193; **Toffee** owned by the Hopkins family: 133br, 236b; **Wallace** owned by Charlene Taylor: 18tr; **Walter** owned by Richard and Heather Nuttall: 122l; **Walter** owned by Rachel Williams: front cover tr, 18bl, 35r, 37, 42m & b, 48b, 55t, 59m, 60b, 61r, 69b, 70m, 82m, 85b, 87tl, 101b, 109t, 120m, 138m, 140, 141, 149r, 150, 152, 153, 154, 158, 171t, 174tl, 178t, 187b, 213t, 216t, 228l; **Widgeon** owned by Sharon Winkler: 104, 132, 159, 162t, 167t; **Wilhelm** owned by Anna Richardson: 182t, 186b; **Willy** owned by Kathleen and Joe: 35bl, 49, 62, 77b, 93; **Wolfgang** owned by Anna Richardson: 182b; **Yogi** owned by Abbie Evans: 41t, 58l, 65t, 115t, 228r; **Zack** owned by Donna Anglim: 51, 120b, 123b, 126, 128t; **Zigzag** owned by Jill Dyer: 138tr, 139t; **Zoey** owned by Donna Anglim: 51, 120b, 128t.

Picture credits *continued*

I am also very grateful to the following for providing images for inclusion:

Archie's workshop: 185, 186t

Charlotte Baldwin for sharing a group photo on behalf of Dedicated to Dachshunds with IVDD: 214b

Sean Cameron Photographic: 182b

Dachshund Health UK: 195t, 240

Eddie's Wheels: 189, 192m

Barbara Houlding GradDipPhys, MScVetPhys, MCSP, FIRVAP, MRAMP, ACPAT Chartered Physiotherapist & Veterinary Physiotherapist for images shared in association with K9HS Courses: 199, 200, 201, 202t & b, 203m & b

Dr Heike Kopac-Pickering: 209

KRUUSE: 92, 113br, 121

Tessa Lewis PGCert, MIRVAP, MCHA and Charlie Nelson MSc, MIRVAP, NAVP, MCHA for sharing photos taken at Cotswold Dog Spa: 203t, 204, 205t

Dr Mark Lowrie (European & RCVS Specialist in Veterinary Neurology) for sharing images from Dovecote Veterinary Hospital: 25

Graham Parker of Ginger and Black Photography: 241t

Paw Prosper – Help 'Em Up Harness: 75tr, 79b

rawpixel: 129t

Dr Ann Tryssessoone: 22b, 102l, 108, 138m, 187m, 198t, 234

Sharon Winkler BSc (Hons) Ost, PGCert (Registered Osteopath & Small Animal Physiotherapy) for sharing the following images: 66t, 82b, 104, 132, 159, 162t, 167t

Foreword by Ian Seath BSc (Hons)

Intervertebral disc disease (IVDD) is undoubtedly the most significant health issue affecting dachshunds, a breed my wife and I have owned and lived with since 1980. Over the years, I have led and been involved in many dachshund health projects as a breed club committee member and chairman of the UK Dachshund Breed Council. I am also a trustee of Dachshund Health UK (dachshundhealth.org.uk) a registered charity that supports research, education and health projects in our breed. In addition to my day-job as a management consultant, I am a Director of The Kennel Club and a member of their Neurology Working Group.

We have been very fortunate in our time owning dachshunds only to have had a few dogs affected by IVDD but, when it happens, it is extremely distressing. Signs can range from relatively mild pain that resolves with rest and medication, to life-changing paralysis that requires surgery or can result in euthanasia. It's also important to remember that dachshunds aren't the only breed to suffer from IVDD; other short-legged breeds are also affected, as well as bigger dogs, albeit for different reasons.

Having worked with Marianne on various projects over recent years, I am delighted that she has found time to write a book which is such a positive addition to the thinking and knowledge on IVDD. This book will be of immense practical value to owners and vets. Until now, there hasn't been a definitive guide such as this book, written for owners of dogs with IVDD. There are numerous websites and online support groups catering for those whose dogs are affected by IVDD but it can be hard for an owner who is incvitably stressed, to find the information they need quickly. Information provided on the internet also comes with its challenges because so much appears to be anecdotal advice, rather than being based on reliable veterinary evidence.

The book is filled with down-to-earth advice drawn from Marianne's experience as a vet and as a specialist in canine rehabilitation. It's a practical handbook, written for lay people. Ordinary dog owners will quickly find the answers to commonly asked questions about the signs and symptoms of IVDD, how their vet will make a diagnosis and the main treatment options available. Whatever course of treatment is chosen, recovery from IVDD can be a long and challenging process, both for the owner and their dog. Marianne carefully explains how to cope with a recovering dog, not just in terms of rehabilitation techniques but also the emotional challenges that owners will face.

Having seen Marianne's approach to consulting and treatment first-hand, I know how skilled she is at connecting empathetically with pet owners and giving them the skills and confidence to support their dog through weeks or months of recovery. It's impossible to replicate that simply by reading a book, but I'm sure everyone who does read this handbook will get a strong sense of Marianne's passion and commitment to help improve the lives of dogs with IVDD.

Contents

Introduction

Author's note

Dachshunds, French bulldogs and some other breeds are prone to back and neck trouble. At its worst, this can be catastrophic. Some dogs lose all use of their legs. Others can still walk but are uncomfortable and unsteady on their feet.

Having worked as a vet and physiotherapist for many years, I have found IVDD to be one of the most distressing conditions both for dogs and for their owners. Some tell me that they feel completely overwhelmed by the experience of seeing their dog suddenly collapsed, or mobile but in great pain. Recovery is often possible, but it requires attention to detail in the dog's home care.

> **NAMING THE PROBLEM: 'DISC EXTRUSION' AND 'IVDD'**
>
> Dachshunds and certain other breeds tend to get a type of back or neck issue called a **disc extrusion**.
>
> This is a type of **IVDD**, which stands for intervertebral disc disease
>
> Some people casually refer to a disc extrusion as a 'slipped disc'. But this is misleading, as the disc does not slip out of position. Instead, think of it as a 'ruptured disc'.
>
> → **For more explanation and a list of affected breeds see Chapter 1: 'What is IVDD'.**

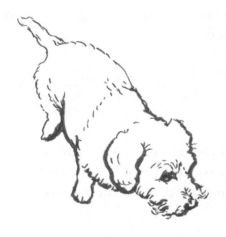 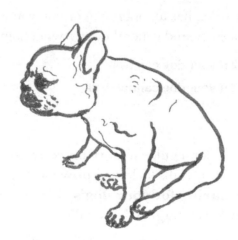

Getting back on all four paws

This home handbook includes practical advice on helping your furry friend through recovery, from first aid to diagnosis, and from treatment to long-term care. Use this in conjunction with talking to your own vet.

❖ **For dogs having spinal surgery**: use this book to prepare yourself for their homecoming and for home care advice.

❖ **For dogs recovering without surgery**: use this book to guide you through their recovery. It includes prompts on when to get extra help from your vet.

Home care advice in this book is also suitable for dogs with some other back or neck conditions, including FCE (fibrocartilaginous embolism, also known as ischaemic myelopathy) and traumatic disc (also known as ANNPE).

How to use this book

Your vet visit

For information on **what to expect from your vet visit**, see Chapter 4. Your vet may offer you the choice between surgical and non-surgical treatment. Find out more in Chapter 6, 'Should my dog have surgery?'

Getting started with your dog's recovery

Whether your dog has an operation or not, you will need to care for them at home. For advice on what to do at what stage and general overviews of home care, see:

→ **Section 2 if your dog can walk**

→ **Section 3 if your dog cannot walk**

How to...

See Chapter 20 for a guide to **setting your dog up in a pen or crate**. This book also includes how-to guides for many skills including **how to sling walk your dog** (Chapter 30), **carrying your dog** (Chapter 31), **caring for your dog's skin during recovery** (Section 9), **home exercises** (Section 10), and **home massage** (Chapter 65).

Some affected dogs lose control of their bladder or bowels. You can find out more about **toileting issues** in Section 8. This includes advice on **how to clean your dog** (chapter 51) and **expressing their bladder** (chapter 49).

Discovering more

To search for information on your chosen topic, go to the **index**. A page number in bold indicates the most complete reference to the subject. Medical and technical terms are defined in the **glossary**.

During your dog's journey of recovery, you may also find the following sections useful: **keeping your dog happy at home during recovery** (Chapter 34), **understanding what your dog is thinking** (Chapter 37), **confidence-building techniques** (Chapter 39), **nutrition** (Section 14), **extra therapies** (Section 15), **your wellbeing** (Section 16) and **recovery on a budget** (Appendix 6).

SECTION 1
Signs to watch for, and what to do

This section explains signs to watch out for:

- Chapter 1: What is IVDD? – an introduction to the condition

- Chapter 2: Spotting the signs of IVDD – knowing when your dog might need help

What to do straight away:

- Chapter 3: **First aid**

Getting diagnosed, and deciding what to do next:

- Chapter 4: What to expect at your vet visit

- Chapter 5: Diagnostic tests

- Chapter 6: Should my dog have surgery?

- Chapter 7: Going for surgery

- Chapter 8: Non-surgical treatment

CHAPTER 1
What is IVDD?

IVDD is the most common back condition in dogs. It can also affect their neck.

IVDD = Intervertebral Disc Disease

Just like people, dogs have discs between the bony vertebrae of their spine. These discs cushion the vertebrae as the dog moves. In dogs with IVDD, the discs degenerate over time and become weaker. A weakened disc may rupture or bulge and start to press on the spinal cord or nearby nerve roots. This can cause pain, difficulty walking, or paralysis.

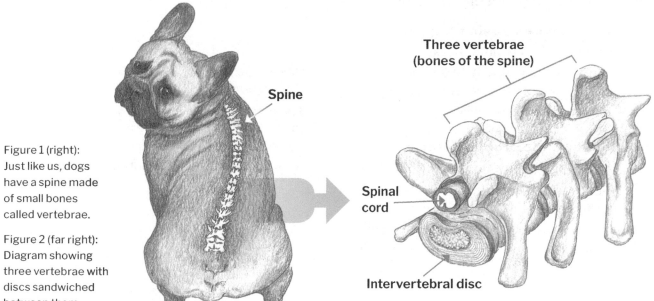

Figure 1 (right): Just like us, dogs have a spine made of small bones called vertebrae.

Figure 2 (far right): Diagram showing three vertebrae with discs sandwiched between them.

Spine

Three vertebrae (bones of the spine)

Spinal cord

Intervertebral disc

Parts of the body affected by IVDD

Back disease (Thoracolumbar disc disease). An abnormal disc in the dog's back can cause:

- back pain
- weak, wobbly or paralysed hind legs and tail
- in severe cases, a loss of bladder and bowel control.

Back problems can block nerve impulses from travelling along the spine between the dog's brain and hind legs. If messages do not get through, the rear part of the body cannot function normally.

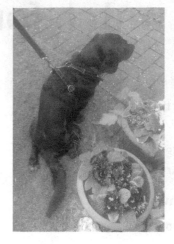
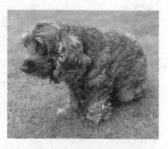

Figure 3 (left): Back disease can cause paralysis of the dog's hind legs.

Figure 4 (above): A dog with neck pain.

Neck disease (Cervical disc disease). An abnormal disc in the dog's back can cause neck pain. These dogs may also have coordination problems involving all four legs. Severe neck disease can also cause irregular breathing and reduced bladder and bowel control.

Types of IVDD, and dogs affected

There are two main types of IVDD:

1. **Disc extrusion**. This tends to affect smaller, short-legged breeds such as dachshunds (see box 1). Signs can be sudden and dramatic.

2. **Disc protrusion**. This is more common in older dogs. It can affect any breed.

Disc extrusion (Hansen type 1 herniation)

When can a disc extrusion happen?
This condition is seen in adult dogs, not in puppies. Problems are usually first noticed between the ages of 4-6 years. Younger adult dogs and older dogs can also be affected.

How fast does the problem start?
Signs of a disc extrusion can start very suddenly, for example with a dog running around playing in the morning, and then unable to walk later the same day. In other cases, the same type of problem may take a few days or a couple of weeks to develop.

DISC EXTRUSION: HOW DO THESE DOGS LOOK?

Milder signs: Back or neck pain with or without a wobbly gait.

Severe signs: Dogs with severe disease cannot walk. Those that are worst affected may also lose control of their bladder and bowels.

→ **Also see Chapter 2, 'Spotting the signs of IVDD'**

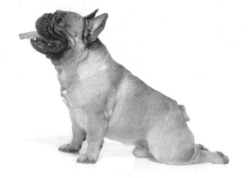

BOX 1: WHICH BREEDS ARE PRONE TO A DISC EXTRUSION?

Dachshunds are at particularly high risk of having a disc extrusion. Around one in five miniature dachshunds, and one in seven standard dachshunds, are affected at some stage in their lives. Some of these dogs are unlucky enough to experience the problem more than once. The breeds listed below are also at much greater than average risk of getting a disc extrusion, and their crossbreeds can also be affected.

Basset, Beagle, Bichon Frise, Cavalier King Charles Spaniel, Chihuahua, Chinese Crested, Clumber Spaniel, Cocker Spaniel (both American and English), Dachshund (miniature and standard), French Bulldog, Lhasa Apso, Maltese, Poodle (miniature and toy), Miniature Schnauzer, Nova Scotia Duck Tolling Retriever, Pekingese, Shih Tzu, Welsh Corgi (Cardigan and Pembroke).

NB: This is not a complete list of breeds that can get a disc extrusion

Dogs carrying the genes for IVDD are called 'chondrodystrophic', meaning 'abnormal cartilage', and they tend to have short legs.

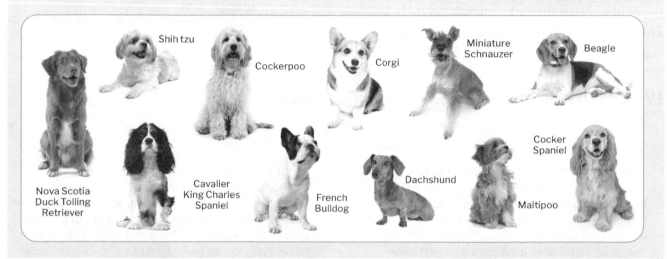

Shih tzu · Cockerpoo · Corgi · Miniature Schnauzer · Beagle · Nova Scotia Duck Tolling Retriever · Cavalier King Charles Spaniel · French Bulldog · Dachshund · Cocker Spaniel · Maltipoo

Some dogs are affected worse than others

BOX 2: GRADES 1 TO 5 FOR DOGS WITH A DISC EXTRUSION

Dogs with IVDD are given a grade from 1 to 5. Those with the mildest signs are grade 1. Dogs with the most severe signs are a grade 5, and are less likely to recover.

CLINICAL GRADE	HOW DOES THE DOG LOOK?			
1	painful			
2	painful	wobbly walking		
3	painful	cannot walk		
4	painful	cannot walk	paralysed legs	Reduced bladder and bowel control	
5	painful	cannot walk	paralysed legs	Reduced bladder and bowel control	cannot feel their toes

Slow onset IVDD: Disc protrusion

Medium to large breeds such as collies and retrievers are more likely to get a different type of IVDD called disc protrusion. This is also sometimes called Hansen Type 2 herniation. Any breed or crossbreed can be affected. Disc protrusion is mainly seen in dogs aged five years and above.

Signs of disc protrusion tend to come on gradually, and may get worse over months or years. During flare-ups, affected dogs may be particularly painful and unsteady on their feet. However, in some dogs, the condition seems to stabilise.

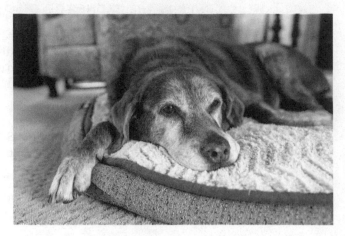

Figure 5: Disc protrusion is most often seen in older dogs.

IVDD: What is happening in the dog's spine?

HOW DOES A DISC EXTRUSION HAPPEN?

In some breeds (see box 1), discs tend to degenerate during the first few years of life. The centre of a degenerated disc can then escape through a split in the outer layer, pressing against the spinal cord and damaging it (figure 6b). This explosion of the disc is called a disc extrusion.

HOW DOES A DISC PROTRUSION HAPPEN?

As part of the natural ageing process, discs in the dog's neck or back wear out or degenerate over time. One or more of these discs can then change shape or gradually bulge (figure 6c). A disc that starts to press on the spinal cord or on other nerves may cause pain, weakness, gradual muscle wasting and, in severe cases, a wobbly walk.

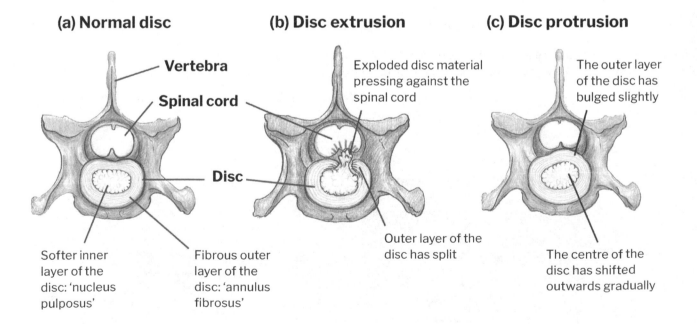

(a) Normal disc

Vertebra

Spinal cord

Disc

Softer inner layer of the disc: 'nucleus pulposus'

Fibrous outer layer of the disc: 'annulus fibrosus'

(b) Disc extrusion

Exploded disc material pressing against the spinal cord

Outer layer of the disc has split

(c) Disc protrusion

The outer layer of the disc has bulged slightly

The centre of the disc has shifted outwards gradually

Figure 6. Diagrams of a normal disc, a disc extrusion and a disc protrusion.

CHAPTER 2
Spotting the signs of IVDD

Early or mild signs

Watch out for early signs of IVDD. They can give you the chance to arrange a veterinary assessment, and to confine your dog to reduce the risk of a problem getting worse. Many dogs appear to be not quite right in themselves for a few hours or days before they lose the ability to walk (see box 3).

BOX 3: EARLY WARNING SIGNS OF IVDD

It is common for dogs to show some of these signs shortly before a severe episode of IVDD:

- Reluctance to walk, jump up or stand upright on hind legs
- Crying or flinching when touched
- Trembling, shaking or panting
- Arched back (figure 7)
- Crying or yelping when picked up

- Refusing to go down a small step or kerb (figure 7)
- Change of mood or temperament (figure 8)
- 'Swollen' or hard abdomen
- Reduced appetite
- Unable to do a full body shake

> If you see two or more of these signs in a dachshund, French bulldog, or other breed prone to IVDD:
>
> 📞 **CALL YOUR VET, and confine your dog just in case.**
>
> → **For more advice, see 'First Aid' (Chapter 3).**

These signs do not confirm that your dog has IVDD, but they are often seen in the early stages of the condition.

For some dogs, these signs of discomfort are as bad as it gets. Other dogs may go on to have more obvious signs of IVDD.

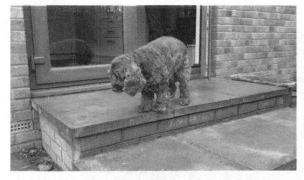

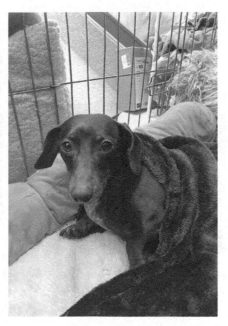

Figure 7 (above): Standing with an arched back, and refusing to go over a step, are typical warning signs of IVDD.

Figure 8 (right): Some dogs are reluctant to move during the early stages of IVDD.

Typical signs of IVDD

BOX 4: TYPICAL SIGNS OF IVDD (DISC EXTRUSION)

Difficulty walking

- Cannot stand or walk, or difficulty doing so.
- Placing paws upside down while standing or walking.
- Staggering gait 'like a drunk person'.
- Legs crossing while walking.
- Dragging their hindquarters.

Other problems

- Pain.
- Hunched posture when standing or sitting.
- Reduced bladder or bowel control: Indoor peeing or pooing.

📞 **CALL THE VET, and confine your dog (see First aid, chapter 3). IVDD is a possibility if your dog is showing any of these signs.**

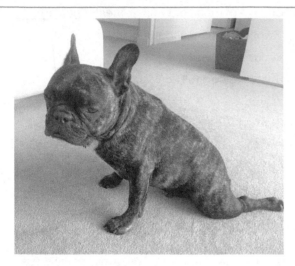

Dragging their hindquarters

Dogs that cannot walk might move by dragging their hind legs along.

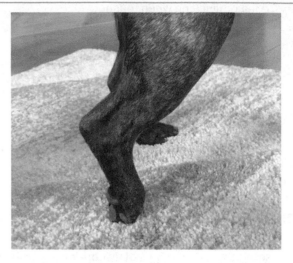

'Knuckling' their paws

It's never normal for a dog to stand or walk with their paws upside-down ('knuckled'). This is often seen with IVDD.

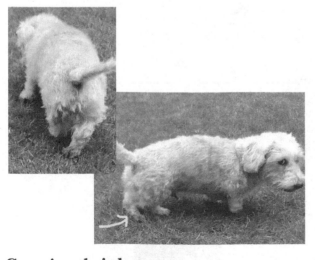

Crossing their legs

Dogs with IVDD may cross their hind paws over when standing and walking.

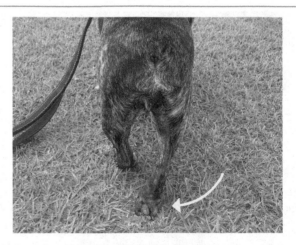

Dragging or scuffing their paws when walking

Affected dogs may drag one or more paws along as they walk.

Some owners remember noticing two or more warning signs of IVDD (see box 3) before their dog's condition becomes obvious. An IVDD episode can then be quite dramatic. A dog could simply wake up one morning unable to walk. If they can walk, then they may be very unsteady on their feet, lurching about, staggering like a drunk person, wobbling and even falling over.

You may find that your dog is slow and reluctant to move. On the other hand, they may try to get about surprisingly quickly, tripping and falling if their legs cannot keep up. Watch out for the signs listed in box 4.

WHICH LEGS ARE AFFECTED?

Which legs are affected?

- Dogs with back issues may knuckle, cross over or drag their hind paws.

- In dogs with neck problems, all four legs may be affected.

Pain

Many dogs with IVDD experience pain, especially in the early stages of the disease. The warning signs of IVDD may continue for a while (see box 3). Pain may also cause:

- distress and screaming
- trembling
- excessive panting
- flinching when touched or lifted
- looking tense in their face.

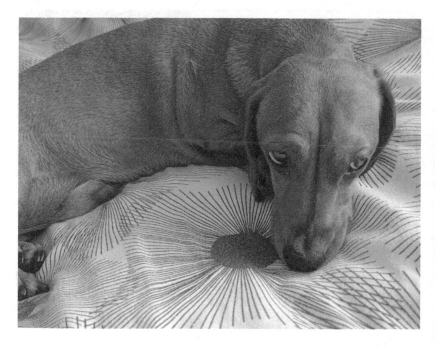

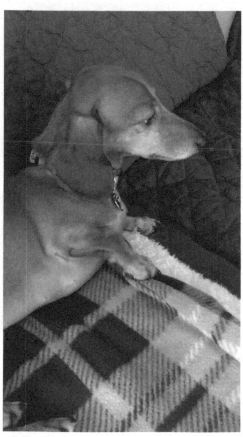

Figure 13 (above): Pain can leave a dog reluctant to move.

Figure 14 (right): This dog was trembling with pain.
→ **Also see chapter 42, 'Is my dog in pain?'**

CHAPTER 3
FIRST AID

Box 5: First aid

If your dog is showing any of the signs described in chapter 2:

CALL THE VET: Ask for the next available appointment.

and

CONFINE YOUR DOG: Use a pen or very large crate if you have one. Remember to include non-slip flooring, bedding and water.

If you don't yet have a crate or pen, or if your dog is a large breed:

✓ Close doors to keep your dog in one room at a time.

✓ Cover any slippery flooring with non-slip matting.

✓ Put a water bowl within easy reach.

✓ Provide bedding at floor level.

✗ Don't let them jump on or off the sofa.

→ **For advice on setting up a pen or crate, see Chapter 20.**

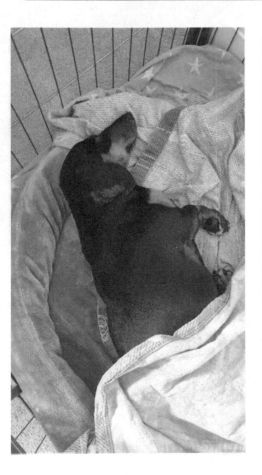

Avoid these activities

✗ **Jumping** on or off the sofa or your bed

✗ **Running**, for example to greet visitors

✗ **Stairs**, going up or down

✗ **Steps**. For small breeds, this includes any doorsteps.

✗ Walking over **slick flooring**

✗ Playing with children or other dogs

 TIP: If your floor is slick, use any rubber-backed matting to make a non-slip area for your dog. Old yoga mats, bathmats or door mats can be useful.

Only give medication that has been prescribed for your dog by their vet. Never give painkillers from your own medicine cupboard unless your vet has specifically told you to do so,

If they need to go outdoors

While waiting for the vet appointment, keep any outdoor toilet breaks very short – no more than five minutes each. Your dog must be on the lead whenever outdoors. If they have a chest harness, attach the lead to the top of this rather than to a collar.

As soon as your dog has had the chance to pee or poo, bring them back in, lifting them over any steps or slick flooring.

Slow them gently from the lead if they try to rush ahead. On the other hand, they might be unable to walk much or at all. Be prepared to stand still with them, or to walk very slowly by their side or just behind.

If your dog must go outdoors, keep them on the lead at all times.

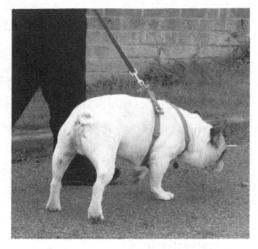

Figure 16: Keep your dog on the lead at all times when outdoors.

🚫 **AVOID THIS...** Don't pull your dog forward to make them go faster. Be patient or carry them.

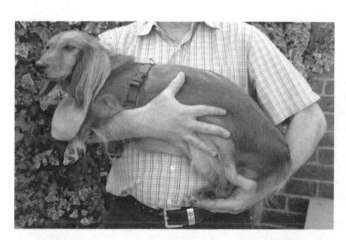

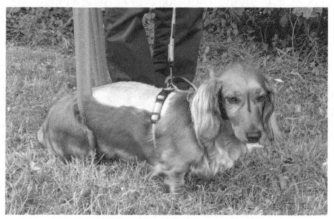

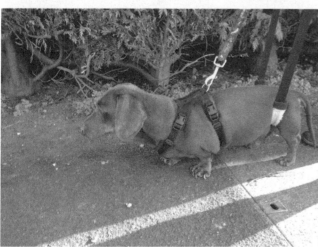

Figure 17 (above left): Carry your dog over any steps or slippery flooring.

Figure 18 (left): If your dog cannot stand or walk without help, support their rear end with a sling.

Figure 19 (above): Improvise if you don't yet have a sling. Loop a scarf or towel under your dog's belly or, for a very small dog, try a fluffy bathrobe belt.

For more details, see:

→ **Setting up the crate or pen, Chapter 20**

→ **Using the lead, Chapter 29**

CHAPTER 4

What to expect at your vet visit

While waiting for your dog's first vet visit

❦ Follow the first aid advice in Chapter 3.

❦ Don't feed your dog within a few hours of the appointment in case immediate surgery is needed.

❦ Check your budget. If your dog has health insurance, how much cover is available per condition?

❦ Make a note of whether your dog pees and poos. This is useful information for the vet.

❦ If time allows, see Chapter 6, 'Decision-making'.

At the clinic

Examination

Your vet will examine your dog and help you decide what to do next. Expect to be asked general questions such as your dog's recent appetite and whether there has been any vomiting. Your answers will help to rule out other conditions.

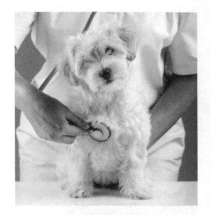

As well as giving your dog a general check-up, your vet might assess their spine for tenderness and check their reflexes, which may include the paw-placing test (see box 8).

BOX 8: PAW PLACING TEST

Figure 20: Vet doing a paw-placing test – The paw is turned upside down (a). A dog with a normal paw placing reflex will immediately replace their paw the correct way up (b).

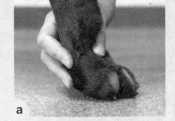
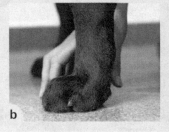

a   b

Advice

Your vet will then tell you what appears to be wrong before advising you. You may be offered one or more of the following:

• Taking your dog home for rest, home care and prescribed medication (see Chapter 8, 'Non-surgical treatment').

• Taking your dog home, but considering referral to a neurologist if the condition gets worse.

• Immediate referral to a neurologist for a scan and surgery (see Chapter 7, 'Going for spinal surgery').

• Admitting the dog for X-rays. This is only useful in a few rather unusual cases (see Chapter 5, 'Diagnostic tests').

• Admitting the dog to the first opinion clinic overnight, before sending home or referring to a neurologist. This can be a sensible option if your clinic has good 24-hour inpatient care.

• Euthanasia (putting the dog to sleep). Don't panic if this option is mentioned. Your vet has a professional responsibility to tell you this is available in some situations (see Appendix 9, 'Thinking about euthanasia').

Part of your vet's job is to help find the best solution for your dog's care within the available budget. Spinal surgery is expensive. Be honest at this stage if you cannot afford this. On the other hand, if you would like your dog to be referred for surgery but it is not offered, suggest it to your vet. They might not have realised that this was an option for you.

What if the diagnosis is uncertain?

If your dog is painful but walking normally, the vet might not be able to tell for sure what is wrong. Some of these dogs might not have IVDD at all, but a different problem such as an upset stomach or a toothache. Follow your vet's advice regarding care and medication. Confine your dog as described in Chapter 10 to help keep them safe just in case this turns out to be IVDD. Arrange a recheck appointment with your vet.

Follow-up

If your dog is referred to a neurologist, ask what to do next. You might have to take them straight to the specialist clinic or bring them home and wait for a phone call.

If your dog is not referred, arrange a follow-up with your own vet. At the recheck, your vet can adjust the pain medicine if needed, and can help your dog if they are having trouble peeing. Check how to contact the clinic's out-of-hours emergency service in case this is needed between appointments.

BOX 8: HELPING YOUR DOG DURING THEIR CHECK-UP

Some dogs are nervous at the vet clinic. Let your vet know if you are concerned that your dog might panic. They can then take this into account and take a gentler approach.

If your dog might growl or snap with close handling, remind your vet to pop a muzzle on them for the hands-on part of the check-up.

If your dog has a chest harness, leave this on during the consultation. You can use it to steady them if they wriggle.

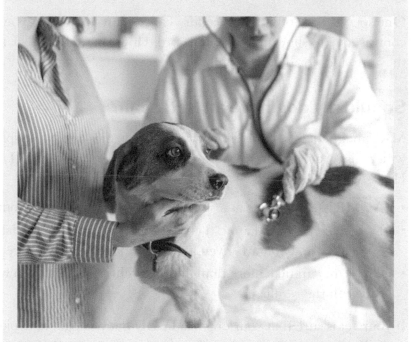

Figure 21: You might be asked to hold your dog during the examination. If so, stand in front of or to one side of them, where they can see you easily. This usually puts the dog more at ease.

CHAPTER 5

Diagnostic tests

If your vet suspects that your dog has IVDD, the problem must be confirmed before surgery using MRI or another advanced imaging technique.

Should my dog have an X-ray?

For dogs showing typical signs of IVDD, the answer is usually "no". Damage to the spinal cord does not show up.

If your vet strongly suspects that your dog has IVDD, spinal X-rays are unlikely to be helpful. An anaesthetic or heavy sedative is needed for the procedure, and surgeons cannot base a spinal operation on X-ray findings unless contrast dye was used.

> **A spinal X-ray does not tell us how badly the dog is affected, or whether they will recover without surgery.**

However, there are a few occasions when it may be useful to X-ray a dog's spine, for example:

- if the dog might have broken their back.
- if the vet suspects infection of a spinal disc ('discospondylitis').
- in healthy dogs, as part of a breed health screening programme (see Appendix 8).

One special type of x-ray procedure called a myelogram can be used to diagnose IVDD. This uses contrast dye to show up the spinal cord. However, MRI or CT are usually used instead now because they are safer for the dog than a myelogram.

Should my dog have an MRI scan?

MRI (magnetic resonance imaging) shows up damage to the spinal cord and can be used to check which disc(s) are involved. Most surgeons therefore do an MRI scan just before operating on the spine. Here's what to expect:

- An MRI scan is done at a specialist centre after referral from your vet.
- Dogs need a general anaesthetic, or sometimes a heavy sedative, for an MRI scan. Follow any guidelines that you are given about withholding food before the appointment.
- The scan can take more than an hour. The specialist team will let you know when to expect a phone call with the results.

If your vet is sure that your dog has IVDD but you plan to avoid surgery, it is often best to avoid a scan. Results would not change how you or your vet care for your dog. Instead, MRI is mainly used for surgical cases, to let the surgeon know exactly where along the spine to operate.

💡 **TIP:** *MRI is expensive.* First check that your budget or insurance policy covers both the cost of MRI and of any expected treatment.

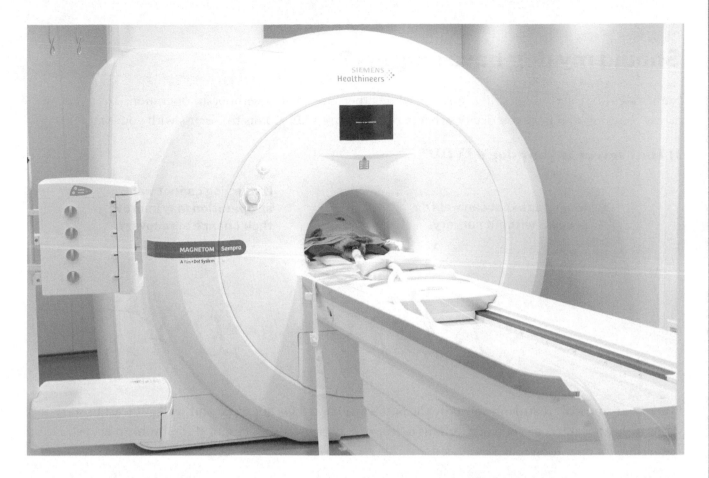

Should my dog have a CT scan?

CT (computer tomography) is another method of imaging the spine. Quicker and sometimes less expensive than an MRI scan, it can be used to diagnose disc herniation and to check which disc(s) are affected. However, some surgeons prefer to use MRI before surgery as this gives more information about damage to the spinal cord.

Figure 22: MRI scan equipment at Dovecote Veterinary Hospital. Above: a dog having an MRI scan. Right: the viewing area where scans are interpreted.

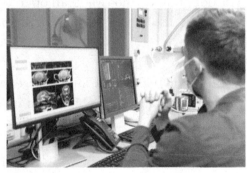

Should my dog have blood or urine tests?

There isn't a blood test to diagnose IVDD. However, your vet might suggest running blood and/or urine tests. Results help to rule out other conditions and can give information about your dog's general health before starting pain medication or surgery.

CHAPTER 6

Should my dog have surgery?

Some dogs are referred for spinal surgery, while others are treated without an operation. Your vet can assess your dog and help you decide what to do. Here are some points to discuss with your vet.

1) How severe is your dog's IVDD?

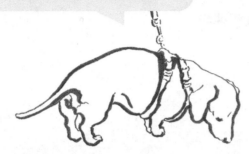

Most dogs that can walk do recover without surgery.

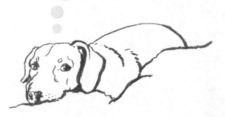

If your dog cannot walk, an operation may improve their chance of recovery.

Good non-surgical treatment is usually the best way forward for dogs that can walk, at least to start with. If the dog starts to get worse or fails to improve over several weeks, or if the problem keeps recurring, an operation may be needed.

For dogs that cannot walk, an operation will give them a better chance of walking again. Some types of operation also reduce the risk of the problem recurring.

2) Cost

Total hospital fees for a miniature dachshund in the UK at the time of writing, including spinal surgery, an MRI scan just beforehand and inpatient care afterwards, are typically £5,000–£10,000 and can be more than this.

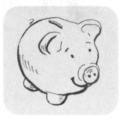

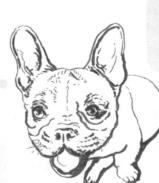

Spinal surgery is so expensive that it is simply out of the question for some dog owners.

⚠ **WATCH OUT!** If your dog is insured, check the small print before surgery. Don't assume that you will be covered for the full cost of treatment. Many policies have limits on what can be claimed for.

→ For more information on the costs involved and insurance, see Appendix 6, 'Recovery on a budget'.

3) Is your dog getting worse and worse?

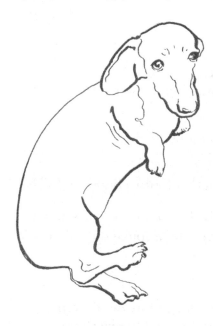

If your dog seems to be getting worse and worse, immediate referral for surgery may improve their chance of recovery.

Mildly affected dogs have the best chance of recovery. However, some appear to have mild, low grade IVDD but then deteriorate over hours or days. If your dog's ability to stand and walk is deteriorating, a prompt operation might stop the problem from getting worse.

We want to prevent the dog's condition from getting so bad that they lose deep pain sensation in their paws. Once deep pain sensation has been lost, chances of recovery following any treatment are much reduced (see Appendix 3).

4) Are you available to care for your recovering dog at home?

Spinal surgery can result in a shorter recovery time. It takes energy and dedication to care for a dog that cannot walk, so a quick recovery would make your life easier.

Having an operation might shorten the recovery time.

For typical non-surgical treatment, you would care for your dog at home from day one.
However, after an operation, a dog with severe IVDD may receive inpatient care for the first week or more. This may put your mind at rest and give you time to get ready for when they come home.

You will need to give your dog special care when they return home whether or not they have had surgery.

5) Your dog's general health

A few dogs have other health issues that could make having an anaesthetic more risky. Your vet can advise you on this.

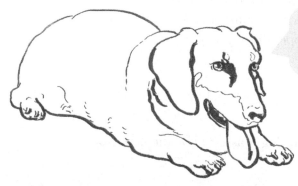

If your dog cannot have an anaesthetic, consider non-surgical treatment instead.

CHAPTER 7

Going for spinal surgery

Why have surgery?

A spinal operation can remove disc material and other debris that is pressing on the spinal cord. In some cases:

- dogs with severe IVDD may be more likely to walk again after an operation.
- operated dogs may recover more quickly than non-operated dogs.
- some types of spinal surgery may reduce the risk of the dog having another future episode of IVDD.

Surgery can also be useful for dogs that have persistent pain due to IVDD. Pain that continues after a good regime of painkillers and lifestyle adjustments may eventually resolve after a spinal operation.

Is surgery urgent?

Prompt surgery may improve chances of recovery for IVDD dogs that cannot walk. Once you make the decision to operate, it is best to do so as soon as possible.

The dogs that need help most urgently are those that are getting worse and worse.

However, results of studies vary: some show that same-day surgery improves chances of recovery while others do not. In most cases, there is time to check your financial situation before going ahead. Even if an operation must be delayed by a few hours or days, take your dog to the vet as soon as possible for assessment and pain medication.

If your dog is finding it more and more difficult to use their legs, a prompt operation may prevent the condition from becoming untreatable. Once deep pain sensation is lost, a dog is classed as having grade 5 IVDD and would have less chance of walking again (see Appendix 3, Clinical Grade Chart)

What does going for surgery involve?

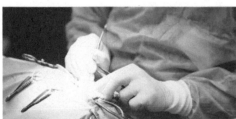

Your first-opinion vet must refer your dog to a neurologist if an operation is needed. The surgeon, anaesthetist and nursing staff all need special skills and experience. Due to the specialist work involved, surgery and hospital care are expensive (see chapter 6, 'Should my dog have surgery?')

Ask your vet if they can recommend a good specialist vet centre within driving distance. A list of referral practices recommended by dachshund owners in the UK is on the UK Dachshund Breed Council website (Appendix 12).

Steps involved in spinal surgery

1. **Referral.** Your vet refers your dog to a specialist centre to see a neurologist. You will need to take the dog to the centre yourself.

2. **Consultation** at the specialist centre. Your dog is assessed by the neurologist.

3. **Admittance**. Your dog is admitted to the hospital for more assessment, imaging and surgery. You will be given paperwork to sign before your dog is admitted. You will either be asked to wait at the centre while your dog has a scan, or to go home and wait for a phone call update.

4. **General anaesthetic**. Your dog is given a general anaesthetic for their scan and operation.

5. **Imaging**. Your dog has an MRI scan or other advanced imaging (Chapter 5).

6. **The operation** takes at least an hour, but may take longer depending on how many discs need to be treated.

7. **Inpatient care**. Your dog is cared for in the hospital after their operation. The number of days spent in hospital depends on how badly they are affected and on how quickly they recover after surgery.

8. **Discharge**. When you come to collect your dog, a nurse or physiotherapist will advise you on how to care for them at home. You may also have the chance to speak to the neurologist.

9. **Home care**. How long you need to care for your dog, and how much you need to do, depend on whether your dog can walk at this point and whether they have bladder and bowel control.

10. **Aftercare appointments**. Over the next few weeks, your dog has one or more follow-up appointments. They may be at the specialist centre or over the phone. You will also need a quick appointment at your local vet clinic to have the surgical staples or stitches removed around ten days after the operation.

Will my dog recover?

Your dog will be in safe hands at a good referral centre. Most dogs that still have deep pain sensation in their hind paws do go on to walk again after surgery.

An operation may make it more likely for a non-walking dog to recover. However, success after spinal surgery is not guaranteed.

In some cases, the spinal cord may have been irreversibly injured at the time of the original IVDD incident. An operation relieves pressure on the spinal cord, but it cannot repair a damaged spinal cord. Many dogs are left with a wobbly walk, some fail to walk again, and occasionally dogs get worse during their time in hospital. Return of bladder and bowel function is also not guaranteed.

In breeds such as dachshunds that are prone to IVDD, signs of the condition can return after treatment. Pain, collapse, or difficulty walking can happen months or years later. Some dachshunds will need to have two or more spinal operations.

Inpatient aftercare

Hospitalisation time varies. In most referral centres, a dog admitted with severe IVDD will stay in hospital for several days after the operation. In hospital, each dog is kept comfortable in a cage. Inpatient care may include an intravenous drip, painkillers, physiotherapy, regular rechecks from the neurology team and help with toileting. If your dog cannot pee, they may have a urinary catheter fitted for a few days. This is a soft plastic tube that takes urine out of the bladder.

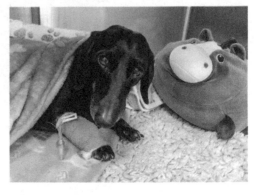

Figure 24: A dog recovering in hospital

Types of spinal operation for IVDD

The surgeon plans the operation based on which disc(s) are affected and the results of the MRI scan.

Decompressive surgery

The surgeon uses special equipment to make holes in one or more vertebrae (bones of the spine). These 'windows' allow the surgeon to see the spinal cord and to remove any disc material and other debris that may be pressing against it. There are three main types of decompressive surgery:

- **Hemilaminectomy.** Used mainly in the thoracolumbar spine (mid-back region), the surgeon accesses the spinal cord from the side. Expect to see sutures or surgical staples on top of the dog's back.

- **Ventral slot.** Used in the cervical spine (neck), the surgeon accesses the spinal cord from underneath. The surgical skin wound will be under the dog's neck.

- **Dorsal laminectomy.** Mainly used for lumbosacral problems (lower back, nearer to the tail). The surgeon accesses the spinal cord from above, and sutures or staples will be on top of the dog's back.

Fenestration

This involves making a hole in a disc and, through that window, scooping out material from the disc's centre. Fenestration does not reduce pressure on the spinal cord. Instead, it is used to help prevent future problems. Discs that have been fenestrated are less likely to herniate in the future. Some IVDD dogs have decompressive surgery of two or more vertebrae and fenestration of several nearby discs.

Understanding your dog's surgical report

When your dog comes home, the surgeon may write a report for you and your vet. This usually includes the date of the operation and the names of any procedures performed. It may also mention where the surgeon operated along the spine. This location is abbreviated (Figure 25).

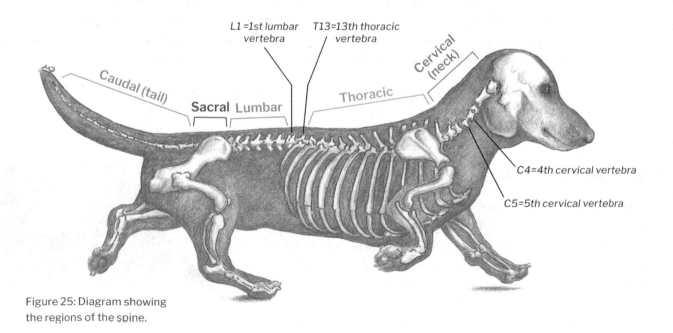

Figure 25: Diagram showing the regions of the spine.

Examples

'**C4-C5 ventral slot**' means that the surgeon has decompressed the spinal cord from underneath, at the level of the 4th and 5th cervical vertebrae (neck bones).

'**T11-T12 left hemilaminectomy**' means that the spinal cord has been decompressed from the left side at the level of the 11th and 12th thoracic vertebrae (this is near the middle of the back).

'**T11-L1 fenestrations**' means that the surgeon has removed the centres of each spinal disc between the 11th thoracic and the 1st lumbar vertebra.

Home care after spinal surgery

After discharge from hospital, you must give your dog any prescribed medication and keep an eye on their surgical wound. You will also need to confine them safely in a crate or pen, and keep them safe when outside this. All toilet breaks must be on the lead.

In the best-case scenario, your dog may return home able to walk quite normally and with excellent bladder and bowel control. However, many dogs, including some considered to be surgical successes, return home initially unable to walk. These dogs need dedicated home care, supported sling walking and exercise therapies before they improve. Some also come home with poor bladder and/or bowel control, so you may need to do extra cleaning and nursing.

For a general overview of home care, see:

→ **Chapter 10 if your dog can walk**
→ **Chapters 12-14 if your dog cannot walk**

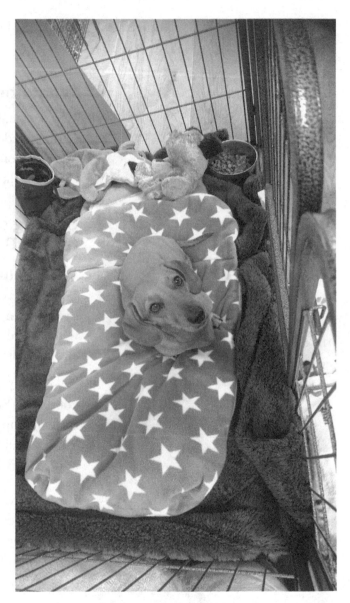

Figure 26: Set up your dog's recovery crate or pen ready for when they get home.

CHAPTER 8

Non-surgical treatment

When to opt for non-surgical treatment

Many dogs with IVDD are treated without surgery, particularly if they have:

- mild signs of IVDD and can walk without falling
- more severe signs, but an operation is out of the question due to cost, availability, or anaesthetic risk.

Non-surgical treatment is sometimes called medical treatment, conservative treatment or conservative management.

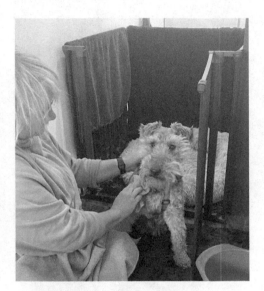

Figure 27: Caring for a dog at home.

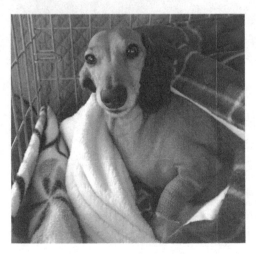

Figure 28: Set your dog up comfortably in a pen or crate (see Section 4, 'Your dog's recovery area').

What does non-surgical treatment involve?

Non-surgical treatment involves similar medication and care to that needed after spinal surgery. It can be time-consuming and may sometimes feel like hard work, particularly if the dog cannot walk and has poor bladder or bowel control.

Getting started with non-surgical treatment for IVDD

Vet appointment

Your own vet can assess your dog, discuss options with you and prescribe medication. They may either send your dog home with advice and prescribed painkillers, or admit them to the clinic for fluids, painkillers and nursing care.

If your dog goes home with you, a next day recheck is often a good idea. Some dogs deteriorate over the first few days. If this starts to happen, your vet might recommend surgical referral. Your vet can also ensure that your dog can pee properly and address this issue if needed.

Back home

Give medication as prescribed, and set your dog up in a recovery pen or crate. How best to care for them at home depends on how badly they are affected. For a general overview of home care, see:

→ Chapter 10 if your dog can walk
→ Chapters 12-14 if your dog cannot walk

How does recovery happen without surgery?

Over time, inflammation goes down. Disc material and other debris that is pressing on the spinal cord may be gradually removed by the body.

Nerve cell recovery. Over the first few weeks, as inflammation settles down, some nerve cells may recover. However, some dogs are left with permanent damage. Nerve cells that are badly crushed or torn will not recover. In that case, the body tries to bridge the gap from one side of the damage to the other so that nerve impulses can get through from the brain again. Spinal nerves on one side of the damaged area can sprout new offshoots that grow slowly across to bridge the damaged area. Over weeks to months, these offshoots eventually connect with other nerve cells (figure 29).

Learning and recovery. The body naturally remodels the nerve sprouts as they grow. Those that appear to help the dog to move are encouraged, while others start to disappear. This remodelling ties in with the learning process. Dogs find that some movement patterns get them to where they want to go, or lead to food reward or praise from an owner. The dog's body strengthens nerve pathways that control these 'successful' movement patterns.

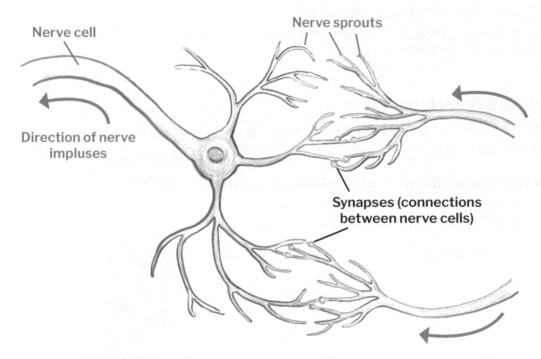

Figure 29: Diagram showing nerve sprouts bridging a gap between two nerve cells

SECTION 2
Dogs that can walk – overview of advice

Section 2 gives general home care guidelines for dogs that can walk.

Chapter 9: What to look for, and what to do next

Chapter 10: Home care for dogs that can walk

Chapter 11: When will my dog recover?

CHAPTER 9
What to look for, and what to do first

KEY POINTS

- 🐾 Dogs with grade 1 and 2 IVDD may have episodes of pain.
- 🐾 Dogs with grade 2 IVDD walk with an unsteady gait.
- 🐾 This could be as bad as it gets, or they might get worse over the next few hours to days. Speak to your vet again if your dog is getting worse.

What do these dogs look like?

Dogs with IVDD are given a grade out of 5. Those able to walk are a grade 1 or 2 (see box 1).

Grade 1 IVDD: Uncomfortable but walking normally
This is the mildest grade of IVDD but is nevertheless unpleasant. These dogs have a painful back or neck. They may:

- cry or flinch when touched or lifted
- tremble, shake or pant.

Each dog shows pain in a different way. Pain may come and go, and your dog might look normal between painful episodes.

→ **See Chapter 43, 'Is my dog in pain?' for advice on recognising when your dog might be uncomfortable.**

Grade 2 IVDD: Walking but wobbly
These dogs walk with a wobbly, staggering gait. The problem only affects the hind legs in dogs with back disease. Dogs with neck disease may also trip or stumble on their front legs.

Many dogs with grade 2 IVDD are also painful at first, as described above for grade 1 IVDD.

BOX 1: IVDD GRADES FOR DOGS THAT CAN WALK

Grade 1: pain only

Grade 2: wobbly walking. These dogs are also usually painful.

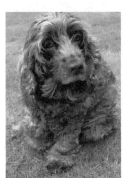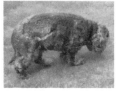

Figure 1a and b: Dogs with grade 1 IVDD can walk quite normally, but are painful and may look hunched.

BOX 2: SIGNS OF GRADE 2 IVDD

- Placing paws upside down while standing or walking
- Staggering gait 'like a drunk person'
- Legs crossing while walking
- Tripping and stumbling

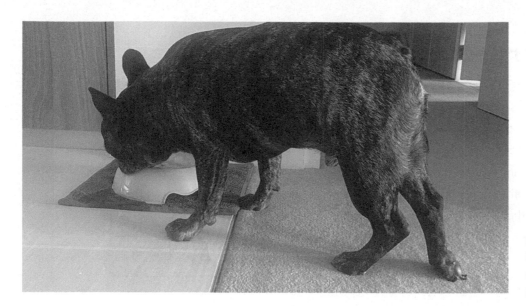

Figure 2: Dogs with grade 2 IVDD are wobbly on their feet and sometimes place their paws upside-down.

What to do first

> **SAFETY ADVICE**
>
> **What to do first**
>
> Call your vet immediately and confine your dog.
>
> → **See 'First aid', Chapter 3.**
>
> Your vet will help you decide what to do next.
>
> → **See Chapter 6, 'Should my dog have surgery?'**

Is this mild IVDD, or warning signs of severe IVDD?

For some dogs, grade 1 or 2 IVDD is as bad as it gets. For others, the pain, with or without the wobbly walk, turn out to be warnings of worse trouble to come. These dogs could potentially get worse and become unable to walk, especially during the first three weeks.

We cannot predict whether a mildly affected dog is about to get worse, even from looking at results of their MRI scan. It's better to be safe than sorry - confine and contain your dog carefully to help keep them safe.

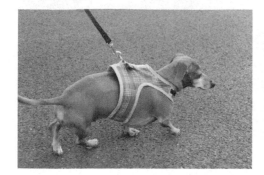

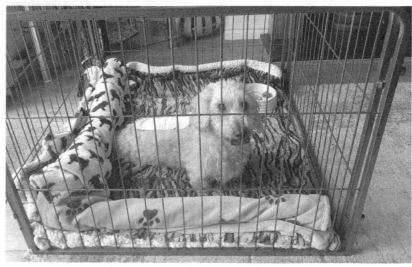

Figure 3 (above): Keep your dog on the lead during recovery, even if they seem ready to do more.

Figure 4 (right): Confine your dog during recovery.

CHAPTER 10

Home care for dogs that can walk

Home care summary

✓ Set your dog up in a crate or pen to keep them safe.

✓ Whenever outside the crate or pen, keep them safe on a lead or in your arms.

- Avoid slippery flooring. Mats are very useful.

✓ Outdoor toilet breaks start at no more than 5 minutes each.

- Keep your dog on the lead whenever outdoors.
- Walk very slowly.

✓ Be patient. Recovery is normally gradual. Don't do too much too soon.

Getting started with home care

Follow the home care advice in this chapter if your dog can walk without a sling. This advice is suitable for dogs with IVDD (non-surgical treatment or home care after spinal surgery) and for dogs with traumatic disc or FCE.

Keeping your dog safe

Set your dog up in a crate or pen. This will prevent them from doing the risky activities listed in box 5. If they are a large breed, room rest may be more appropriate. Check this first with your vet.

→ **See Section 4, 'Your dog's recovery space' for details of choosing and setting up a crate or pen.**

Most dogs should start in an 'Early Rest' crate or pen, and then move to a larger one on the advice of their vet, usually around three weeks into recovery.

→ **See Appendix 4 for a breed chart with recommended crate and pen sizes.**

BOX 5: MY DOG CAN WALK. WHY MUST THEY BE CONFINED?

🐾 To allow any inflammation to go down

🐾 To keep them safe and reduce their risk of getting worse

🐾 For those with a wobbly walk - to help them learn to walk normally again.

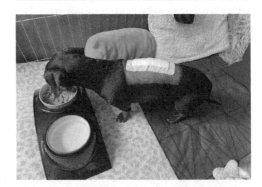

Figure 5: Keep your dog in the crate or pen whenever you are not holding them. They should even eat and drink in there.

Activities to avoid during recovery

SAFETY ADVICE

Don't let your dog move over:
- slick flooring
- stairs
- steps. For small breeds, this includes doorsteps.

Avoid:
- jumping – for example, on or off sofas
- falls – don't leave your dog on a sofa, bed or other furniture

Don't let them play with:
- other dogs
- balls
- toys that they might shake violently.

The daily routine

Your dog's routine should include toilet breaks on the lead outdoors, mealtimes in the crate or pen, medication doses, and at least one expected quiet time per day during which they should not expect attention from you. If your dog usually enjoys daily close contact with you, then you can include one or two periods of 'together time' when you can sit quietly and safely together on the floor, with your hand on their harness (Chapter 32).

→ **For an example routine, see Appendix 1, Routine 1 'Movers and Improvers'**

Outdoor time

Outdoor time must all be on the lead to start with. Start with no more than five minutes at a time, including any time spent standing around and sniffing. Take your dog outdoors as often as is needed for toileting, which could be up to 7 times per day.

Walk very slowly with your recovering dog. They should be walking, not trotting, during early recovery. This will feel much slower than you are used to moving, especially if they are a small or short-legged breed.

→ **See Chapter 29, 'Using the lead' for advice on how to hold the lead. A two-handed lead technique gives best control.**

Getting your dog comfortable

Start by visiting your vet. They can assess your dog and prescribe painkillers. Once back home, there is plenty more that you can do to help your dog feel better. This includes checking that the crate or pen are comfortable, handling your dog gently, and adjusting their routine and activity levels. For more details, see:

→ **Chapter 44, 'Caring for your dog during a pain episode'**

→ **Chapter 45, 'Help! My dog is on painkillers but is still painful'**

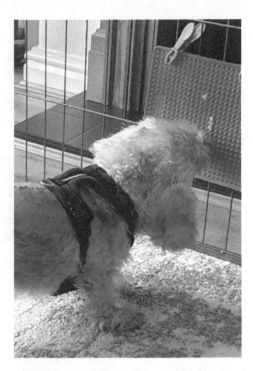

Figure 6 (left): To help keep your dog occupied, feed at least part of their daily ration from safe food dispensing toys such as this lick mat (Chapter 35).

Figure 7 (below): If your dog stops and stands still, stop with them until they get going again.

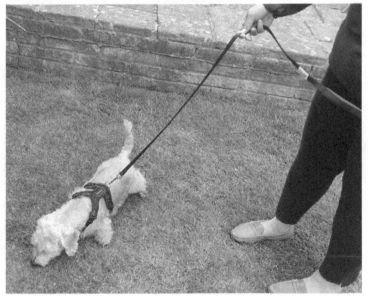

Building up your dog's exercise

Only increase your dog's outdoor time once your vet is happy for you to do so. Each dog recovers at a different rate. Don't increase your dog's walks if they are still having bouts of pain, or if they are very wobbly on their feet.

Increase the length and complexity of your dog's walks very gradually.

→ **For further details, see Chapter 70, 'Building up their walks'**

Gradually add on-lead exercises to your dog's walk as they recover (see box 7), checking with your vet as needed. These will improve your dog's strength, coordination and paw position sense ('proprioception').

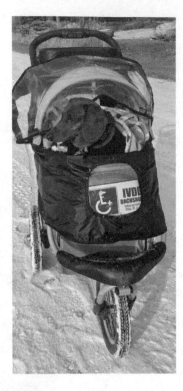

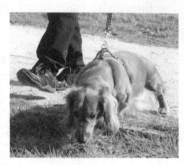

Figure 8 (left): A pushchair is useful while increasing your dog's walks. Watch your dog for signs of tiring (Chapter 70), and rest them for a while if needed.

Figure 9 (below): Add small level changes once your dog is ready.

BOX 7: EXERCISES ON HARNESS AND LEAD FOR DOGS THAT CAN WALK (GRADE 1 AND 2 IVDD).

WHEN TO START	EXERCISE	CHAPTER REFERENCE
Week one of recovery	Three, two, one, stop	Ch. 61, Starter lead exercises, no. 1
	Mats track	Ch. 61, Starter lead exercises, no. 2
Once they are ready Introduce these one at a time once your vet is happy for you to do so. Your dog should first be pain-free and able to walk quite normally on level ground.	Varying the lead pressure	Ch. 63, Further lead exercises, no. 1
	Walking slowly over twigs, uncut grass and bumpy ground	Ch. 70. Building up your dog's walks
	Walking up a short uphill slope	Ch. 70. Building up your dog's walks
	Stepping over a hosepipe	Ch. 63, Further lead exercises, no. 2
	Careful stepping over a low kerb	Ch. 70. Building up your dog's walks
	Trot for a count of five	Ch. 63, Further lead exercises, no. 3
	Walking over a low doorstep	Ch. 63, Further lead exercises, no. 4

Increasing their freedom

It takes time for the body to heal. A relapse is possible if you let your dog do too much too soon.

❧ If your dog has had an operation, follow your surgeon's advice regarding when to let them out of their crate and off the lead.

❧ If your dog has not had an operation, don't allow them to go off-lead or to wander outside their crate or pen for at least six weeks. The start point for this is their most recent episode of pain or weakness. Check first with your vet.

Once your dog starts to come out of their crate or pen, build up their freedom gradually.

→ **For more details, see Chapter 71, 'Starting to come out of the crate or pen'.**

CHAPTER 11
When will my dog recover?

- ❀ Full recovery may take some time. Be patient, and keep in touch with your vet.
- ❀ Each dog is different. Some dogs will recover faster than others.

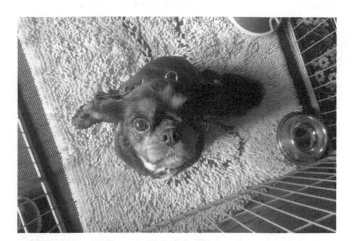

Figure 10: Have your dog complete their prescribed rest period, even if they are feeling much better.

Recovering from pain

Quick recovery

Some dogs start to feel better within a week of starting painkillers, crate rest, and a good 'Movers & Improvers' routine (see Appendix 1). They could feel quite normal again by three to four weeks, even without having had spinal surgery.

Slower recovery

Each dog recovers at their own rate. Some need four weeks or more of painkillers and reduced activity before they start to feel much better.

If your dog is still having bouts of pain after their initial painkiller prescription, then do not increase their walk length or speed, or let them wander loose outside their crate. Instead, ask your vet's advice. They may need to assess your dog and adjust the medication.

Recovering from a wobbly gait

Most dogs get at least a little steadier on their feet within the first two weeks of starting crate or pen rest and starting a good lead technique (Chapter 29).

Time taken to walk normally again varies greatly. Though some grade 2 dogs walk normally by six weeks into recovery, many others are still slightly unsteady on their hind paws by this stage. They might scrape their claws slightly when they walk, and their hindquarters might sway a little when they stand.

Full recovery could take four months or more, and some dogs are left with a slightly wobbly walk long term.

Box 8: What to do if pain continues

Contact your vet if pain is very severe despite good care and medication, or if it is still a significant problem at 6-8 weeks into recovery. Referral to a neurologist may be needed.

Some dogs seem to improve, but then their pain restarts. Overactivity on 'good' days can lead to a cycle of improvement and setbacks. To avoid this, confine your dog, and use their harness and lead to keep them safe whenever outside their crate or pen.

→ **For troubleshooting advice, see Chapter 45, 'Help! My dog is on painkillers but is still in pain'.**

Box 9: Watch out for setbacks

Your dog should look stronger and more stable each week. However, it is normal for there to be recovery 'plateaus' during which they don't improve for a few days.

If your dog seems to be getting worse at any stage, confine them carefully and ask your vet's advice.

→ **For further details, see Chapter 75, 'Is my dog having a relapse?'**

SECTION 3
Dogs that cannot walk – overview of advice

Section 3 is an overview of advice for dogs that cannot walk,

Chapter 12: Getting started with home recovery

Chapter 13: Top tips for learning to walk

Chapter 14: Building up their strength

Chapter 15: When will my dog walk again?

Follow the home care advice in this section if your dog cannot walk without a sling. This applies to dogs with:

- IVDD (non-surgical treatment or after spinal surgery)

- traumatic disc (= ANNPE)

- FCE (= ischaemic myelopathy or 'spinal stroke')

What to do first

Call your vet immediately and confine your dog.

→ **See 'First aid', Chapter 3.**

Your vet will help you decide what to do next.

→ **Also see Chapter 6, 'Should my dog have surgery?'** if your vet suspects that they may have IVDD.

CHAPTER 12
Getting started with home recovery

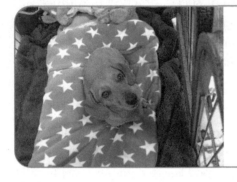

KEY POINTS

- 🐾 **Set your dog up in a crate or pen** during recovery.

- 🐾 **Set up a routine at home** for your dog including food, medication, water, regular outdoor toilet breaks with sling support, cleaning them and expressing their bladder if needed.

- 🐾 **Keep in touch with your vet** and ask their advice as needed.

Preparing for recovery

Home care for a dog that cannot walk may feel like a challenge. They must be confined indoors and supported with a sling during each outdoor toilet break. Some dogs also have poor bladder or bowel control for a while and need extra cleaning. In the early days, your dog will need someone at home to keep an eye on them.

You'll need some basic equipment to get started, including a crate or pen, bedding, harness and sling.

→ See Appendix 2 for a suggested shopping list.

BOX 1: BEFORE YOUR DOG COMES HOME

If your dog is starting their recovery in hospital, set their recovery area up ready for them to come home. Check the following with your vet before your dog returns home:

- Can they pee on their own, or will you need to express their bladder?

- Do you need to buy special padding such as a mattress for your dog, or will basic padding be suitable? (Chapter 22)

- Will you have to turn your dog? (Chapter 55)

- Do they need an Elizabethan collar (cone) and if so will the hospital provide one?

Home care

Keeping your dog safe

Rushing around could make your dog's back or neck problem worse. Don't be caught out. They might surprise you by lurching or scrambling about unexpectedly, for example in response to the post arriving.

Set your dog up in a crate or pen. This will prevent them from doing the risky activities listed in box 3. For large breeds, room rest may be more appropriate. Check this first with your vet.

→ **See Section 4, 'Your dog's recovery space' for details of choosing and setting up a crate or pen.**

Your dog should start in an 'Early Rest' crate or pen, and then move to a larger one when they are ready, usually around three weeks into recovery.

→ **See Appendix 4 for a breed chart with recommended crate and pen sizes.**

Box 3: Activities to avoid during recovery

SAFETY ADVICE

Keep your dog off slippery flooring – put down mats if needed.

Avoid:
- stairs
- steps. For small breeds, this includes doorsteps.

Avoid:
- trying to jump – for example, on or off sofas
- falls – don't leave your dog on a sofa, bed or other furniture

Don't let them play with:
- other dogs
- balls
- toys that they might shake violently.

Don't let your dog drag or scoot themselves across the floor.

BOX 2: WHY MUST MY DOG BE CONFINED?
- To allow any inflammation to go down
- To keep them safe and reduce their risk of getting worse
- To stop them learning the habit of dragging themselves about. This would make it harder for them to learn to walk.

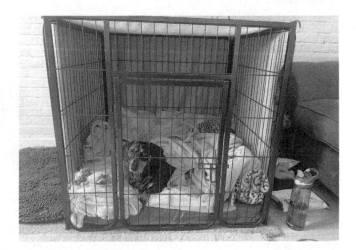

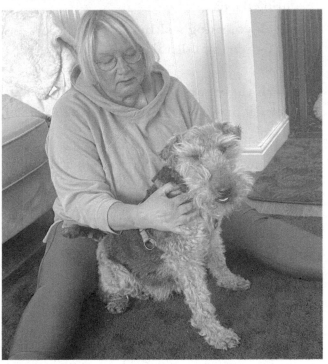

Figure 2 (top): A pen suitable for early recovery

Figure 3 (above): Whenever your dog is outside their crate or pen, keep hold of them so they don't drag themselves about.

Getting your dog comfortable

Prescribed painkillers from your vet will get your dog off to a good start. There is also plenty that you can do at home to help them feel better.

→ See Chapter 44, 'Caring for your dog through an episode of pain'.

The daily routine

Set up a regular routine for your dog so they know what to expect.

The basics

Include the following in their routine:

✓ **mealtimes** in the crate or pen

✓ **medication** doses as prescribed by your vet

✓ **sling-supported toilet breaks** on the lead outdoors (see box 5).

✓ top up their **drinking water** often and, if they cannot move about easily, bring the bowl to them every couple of hours during the day.

✓ **check your dog's skin** each day for sores or other damage (Chapter 54).

✓ **check their surgical wound** each day until it has healed if they have had an operation (Chapter 33).

Some paralysed dogs need turning at least every four hours to help prevent sores. Ask your vet whether you need to do this (see Chapter 55, 'Avoiding pressure sores').

For dogs with poor bladder or bowel control

Your dog may have accidents indoors, so be prepared to wipe them clean or sponge-bathe them and to change their bedding as often as needed.

→ See Section 8, 'Toileting issues'

If your dog cannot yet pee on their own, your vet may ask you to express their bladder. This is usually needed three times daily.

→ See Chapter 49 for advice on expressing your dog's bladder

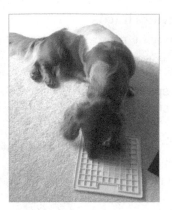

Figure 4: To help keep your dog occupied, feed at least part of their daily ration from food dispensing toys (Chapter 35).

BOX 4: EXAMPLE ROUTINES

See Appendix 1 for suggested routines, and adjust them to suit your dog's needs.

- Use **Routine 2 (Learners)** if your dog cannot walk but is clean indoors

- Use **Routine 3 (Leaky Learners)** if your dog cannot walk and has poor bladder or bowel control

BOX 5: OUTDOOR TIME

Outdoor time must all be on the lead to start with. Support your dog with a sling. Take them outdoors as often as is needed for toileting, usually 3-7 times per day. Have them on their feet for no more than five minutes at a time, including any time spent standing around and sniffing.

→ For advice on how to use the sling, see Chapter 30

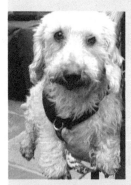

Figure 5 (left): Carry your dog to reach a suitable patch of grass for toileting.

Figure 6 (below): Use the lead and harness to slow your dog's front end.

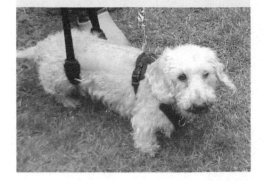

Optional extras

If your dog usually enjoys daily close contact with you, you can include one or two periods of 'together time' when you sit quietly and safely together on the floor, with your hand on their harness (Chapter 32).

You can also start taking them on short pushchair rides from around two weeks into recovery (Chapter 36).

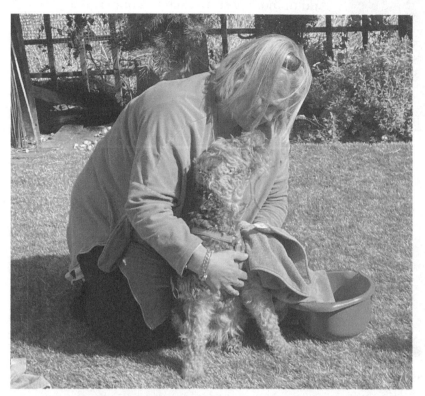

Exercises

Exercises will help your dog to get stronger and improve their coordination. Starter exercises are useful from the first week of recovery. Add them in once you feel ready:

Standing practice (Chapter 58). Support your dog for ten seconds in a standing position, on all four paws. Then lower them gently to the floor.

'Three, two, one, stop' (Chapter 61, exercise 1). When sling-walking your dog, use the lead to bring them gently to a standstill. Correct their paw position if needed, then let them move forward again.

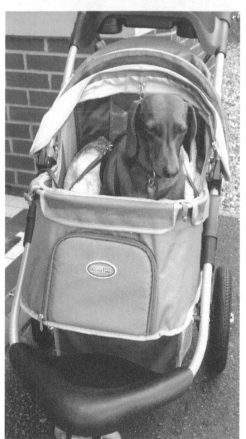

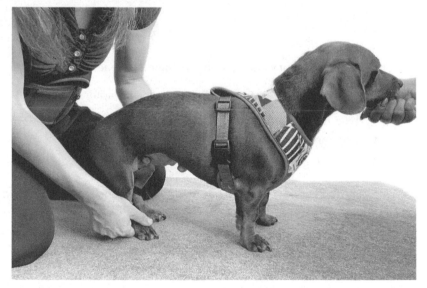

Figure 7 (top): Sponge-bathing.

Figure 8 (left): Pushchair rides can be included in the daily routine.

Figure 9 (above): Standing practice.

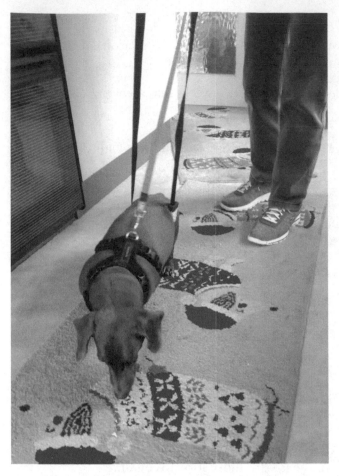

Figure 10: A mats track – use the lead to keep your dog slow, and the sling to support their hindquarters.

Mats track (Chapter 61, exercise 2). Add this in once you and your dog are confident with sling-walking. Walk your dog slowly over a line of non-slip mats.

Add in more posture exercises one by one (Chapter 59) once you are confident with standing practice and are ready to do more. If you're not sure, ask a physiotherapist to assess your dog and to check what you are doing with them.

Massage

Massage, range of movement and sensory touch can be useful for these dogs. However, they are not top priorities during home care. Miss them out if you are feeling overburdened, or if your dog dislikes close handling.

See Chapter 64 for a general guide to touch techniques along with a suggested order in which to learn these. Suggested massage routines are shown in box 6. If in any doubt, have a physiotherapist assess your dog and show you exactly what to do.

BOX 6: SUGGESTED HOME MASSAGE ROUTINES

For a dog that cannot walk but can feel their legs (back disease: grade 3-4 IVDD)

1. Position your dog comfortably on their side (Chapter 64)
2. Stroking massage (effleurage) of body and hind legs (Chapter 65)
3. Hind leg range of movement (ROM) (Chapter 66)
4. More stroking massage of body and hind legs

For a dog that cannot walk and has no deep pain sensation (back disease: grade 5 IVDD)

1. Position your dog comfortably on their side (Chapter 64)
2. Stroking massage (effleurage) of body and hind legs (Chapter 65)
3. Hind leg range of movement (ROM) (Chapter 66)
4. Sensory touch work: stroking massage of body and hind legs, now using fabric or other textured material (Chapter 67)
5. Paw pad sensory touch work (Chapter 67)
6. Pinch withdrawal exercise (Chapter 68)
7. A few strokes of stroking massage (body and hind legs) to finish

CHAPTER 13
Top tips for learning to walk

- **Don't let your dog drag themselves about.** This makes it harder for them to learn to walk.
- **Avoid slippery flooring.** Mats are useful.
- **Use the harness, lead and sling with good technique** to give your dog's legs a better chance to step (see Chapters 29 and 30)
- **Little and often is best.** These dogs tire quickly.
- **Consider what motivates your dog.** Use this to help get them moving.

Setting your dog up for success

Starting to walk again involves a learning process. Adjust their lifestyle to make it easier for them to learn to stand and walk, so they don't learn to drag themselves about instead.

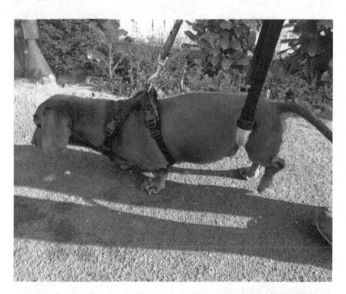

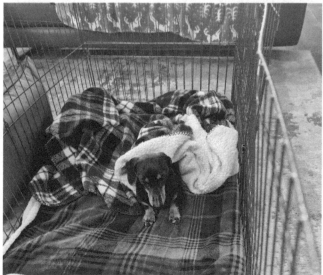

BOX 7: HELP YOUR DOG TO AVOID DRAGGING AND SCOOTING THEMSELVES ABOUT

Weak or paralysed dogs soon learn to drag or scoot themselves about. Unfortunately, dragging and scooting cause problems long term: getting from A to B by dragging or scooting can make it harder for dogs to learn to walk properly. They're also inefficient and cause skin damage and sores.

If we're not careful, dragging or scooting become a dog's new habitual way of moving. Reduce your dog's opportunity to learn to drag or scoot:

- ✓ **Support them up on all four paws** when outdoors: use a lead, harness and sling.
- ✓ **Set them up in a crate or pen** (or a recovery room for large dogs)
- ✓ **Cover any slippery flooring** with non-slip matting

Figure 11 (above left): Support your dog's rear end with a sling. This puts them in a good position to learn to walk instead of learning to drag themselves along.

Figure 12 (left): Confine your dog to a crate or pen so they cannot drag themselves across the room.

Learning through exercises

Simple, safe exercises help the learning process along.

Learning to walk is a challenge. Exercises break this down into small chunks that your dog can manage.

Early exercises include supporting the dog in sitting, standing or walking positions, gradually training them to hold these positions, and helping them to move from one position to another.

→ **See chapter 57 for advice on getting started with exercises.**

Repeat a short exercise through the week to help your dog learn. Little and often is best.

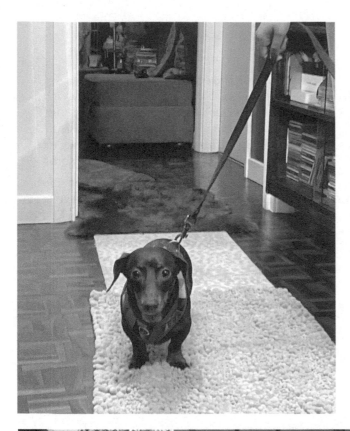

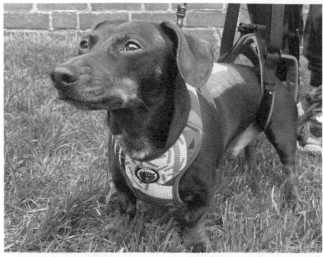

Figure 13 (above): Use a harness and lead to slow down your dog's front end, so their hind paws have a chance to stand or step.

Figure 14 (left): Cover slippery flooring with mats to make it easier for your dog to stand and walk.

Figure 15 (below): Use little rewards during exercise sessions to keep your dog motivated.

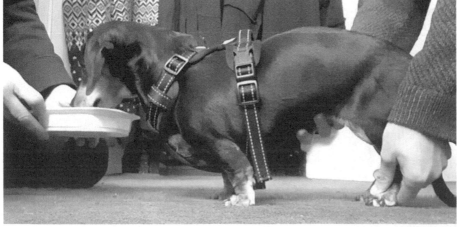

Helping your dog to get motivated

Dogs will only learn to walk if they want to get somewhere. Consider what motivates your dog, and try to include this in their routine.

WHAT DOES YOUR DOG LOVE?	HOW TO MOTIVATE YOUR DOG
Food	Sling-walk them along a food trail. Take care – use the lead to keep them slow.
Favourite person	Walk your dog towards that person over a mats track or outdoors
Favourite corner of the garden	Place them on the ground a few feet or metres from that corner, and let them walk towards it.
Resting in their pushchair	Take them out of the pushchair briefly, place them on the ground a few feet or metres away, and let them walk towards it, with sling support. Reward them with a pushchair ride as soon as they reach it.
Going back indoors	Carry your dog and place them on the lawn, facing the house. Let them walk, with sling support, towards the house.

🚫 **TAKE CARE:** Your dog might have a sudden burst of enthusiasm, especially if food is involved. Use the lead to keep them slow, and don't let them stay on their feet for longer than your vet has advised.

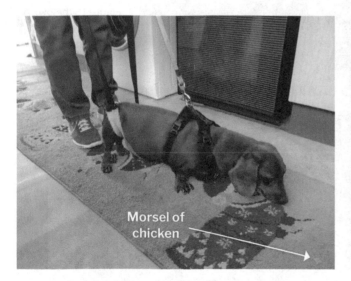
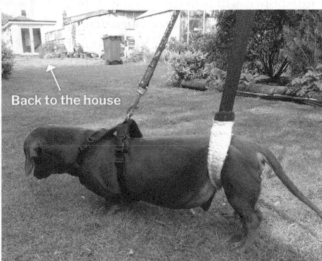

Morsel of chicken

Back to the house

Figure 16a and b: Your dog will make their best walking attempts when going towards something that they love.

CHAPTER 14

Building up their strength

Learning to walk is a gradual process

It is unusual for a paralysed dog to simply get up and start walking. They must first learn to stand and to push off from the floor. While your dog learns how to walk, watch for little signs of success over several days or weeks (see Chapter 15).

> **Don't expect it all to happen at once!**

Remember...
Your dog must learn to stand before they can walk.

And they should learn to walk slowly before starting to trot or run.

Learning to stand

Learning to stand is an important milestone on the recovery journey.

A non-slip standing area in your dog's crate or pen will help them achieve this. The crate or pen floor area can usually be increased to Late Rest size from around three weeks after injury or surgery (check first with your vet). This will give your dog a chance to stand and take some first steps.

→ **See Appendix 4, 'Crate and pen sizes.'**

Posture exercises will also help your dog learn to stand. Start with 'Standing practice' (Chapter 58) and add in further exercises gradually once you and your dog are confident with this (Chapter 59).

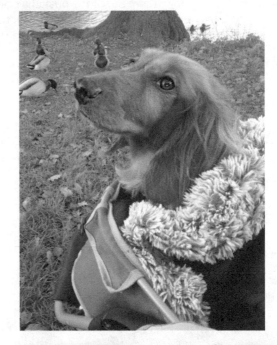

Figure 17 (left): A pushchair is very useful during recovery. Let your dog walk for just a few minutes, with sling support if needed, then return them to the pushchair for a rest.

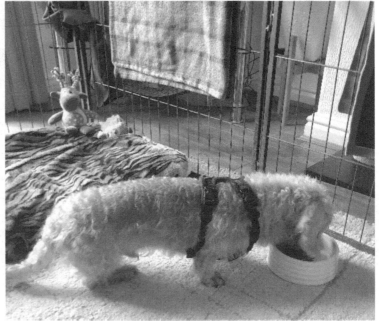

Figure 18 (below): A Late Rest pen. From around three weeks, give your dog a non-slip standing area next to their bed.

Learning to walk without a sling

Help your dog learn to walk without a sling once they are ready. They must first be able to stand and step a little. Some dogs are only strong enough at two or more months into recovery, while others recover much faster and can start as early as week one. Check with your vet if needed.

TOP TIPS

LEARNING TO WALK WITHOUT A SLING

✓ Keep your dog on harness and lead

✓ Walk on the side of their weaker hind leg.

✓ Start by lowering the sling while your dog is standing.

✓ Once you have taken the sling away, aim to have your dog walk a very short distance– no more than 2 metres.

→ See Chapter 63, 'Learning to walking without a sling' for full instructions. For many dogs, it's a gradual process that takes days or weeks to complete.

Once your dog can walk without a sling

To start with, your dog will tire even more quickly than when they had sling support. As soon as they start to get wobbly, rest them for a few minutes in a pushchair or by carrying them. Many dogs can only stand or walk well for up to 60 seconds to start with. Over the next two to three weeks, as their stamina improves, gradually build their walking time back up to 5 minutes.

Many dogs are wobbly on their feet to start with. Help them as follows:

✓ keep them on the lead

✓ walk very slowly

✓ walk just behind and to one side of your dog

✓ walk on the side of their weakest hind leg, if they have one.

→ See Chapter 29, 'Using the lead' for more information.

Building up your dog's walks

Increase the length and speed of your dog's walks very gradually.

→ For further details, see Chapter 70, 'Building up their walks'.

Gradually add exercises to your dog's lead walks as they recover (see box 9), checking with your vet as needed. These will improve your dog's strength, coordination and paw position sense ('proprioception').

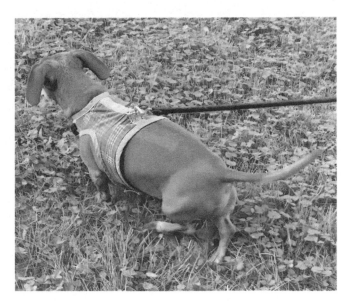

Figure 19: Always keep the lead pointing back from its clip.

BOX 9: EXERCISES ON HARNESS AND LEAD FOR DOGS THAT LOST THE ABILITY TO WALK

WHEN TO START	EXERCISE	CHAPTER REFERENCE
Week one of recovery	Three, two, one, stop	Ch. 61, Starter lead exercises, no. 1
Once you and your dog are confident with sling-walking	Mats track	Ch. 61, Starter lead exercises, no. 2
Once your dog can stand and step a little	Learning to walk without a sling	Ch. 62, Learning to walk without a sling
Introduce these one at a time once your vet is happy for you to do so. Your dog should first be pain-free and able to walk quite normally on level ground.	Varying the lead pressure	Ch. 63, Further lead exercises, no. 1
	Walking slowly over twigs, uncut grass and bumpy ground	Ch. 70, Building up their walks
	Walking up a short uphill slope	Ch. 70, Building up their walks
	Stepping over a hosepipe	Ch. 63, Further lead exercises, no. 2
	Careful stepping over a low kerb	Ch. 70, Building up their walks
	Trot for a count of five	Ch. 63, Further lead exercises, no. 3
	Walking over a low doorstep	Ch. 63, Further lead exercises, no. 4

Increasing their freedom

It takes time for the body to heal. A relapse is possible if you let your dog do too much, too soon.

❧ If your dog has had an operation, don't let them out of their crate or off the lead until your surgeon has assessed them and recommended this.

❧ If your dog has not had an operation, don't allow them to go off-lead or to wander outside their crate or pen for at least six weeks. Many dogs are still unsteady on their feet at this stage and should be confined for longer. Check first with your vet.

Once your dog starts to come out of their crate or pen, build up their freedom gradually.

→ **For more details, see Chapter 71, 'Starting to come out of the crate or pen'.**

Your dog's posture after recovery

Some dogs are left with a hunched back after an episode of IVDD. This is not normally associated with pain, and a hunched appearance long term is usually nothing to worry about. In many cases, the hunch reduces gradually over several months as the muscle tone returns to normal.

CHAPTER 15

When will my dog walk again?

SUMMARY

- ❧ **Each dog is different.** Some recover faster than others.
- ❧ **Some dogs are affected worse than others.** Grade 5 dogs have less chance of making a full recovery. Your vet can check for this.
- ❧ **Learning to walk is a gradual process.** Be patient, and keep in touch with your vet.

Predicting recovery

Each dog has a different recovery journey. Some are up on their paws again within days, while others take months to learn to walk. Full recovery is not guaranteed. Some dogs don't walk again, and many that are considered to have recovered are left a little unsteady on their feet.

A dog's chances of walking again depend on how badly they were affected. Dogs are graded from 1 to 5, with grade 5 dogs being worst affected and less likely to walk again.

→ **See Appendix 3, 'Clinical grade chart'**

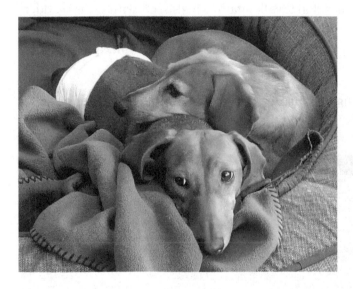

BOX 10: RECOVERY AFTER SPINAL SURGERY

- ✓ How a dog is doing the day *after* their spinal operation can help predict their recovery.
- ✓ Dogs that can make deliberate movements of their legs the day after spinal surgery are expected to take their first steps sooner (average 7 to 10 days) than dogs with paralysed legs (average two to three weeks).
- ✓ If your dog has paralysed legs and they lost deep pain sensation in their toes (Grade 5 IVDD), then they are less likely to recover, and may take a long time to do so.

Grade 3 and 4 dogs

These dogs are unable to walk, but can still feel their toes (box 11). Most of them have the potential to walk again. Those that are going to recover usually start to push up and step within the first month. However, some take three months or even longer to take their first steps.

Grade 5 dogs

These dogs have paralysed legs and no deep pain in their toes. Their chances of walking again are uncertain (see Appendix 3, 'Clinical grade chart').

Grade 5 dogs that do recover usually start walking again within the first three months, though some take much longer than this.

For grade 5 dogs, a promising first sign of recovery is the return of deep pain sensation (box 11). If deep pain sensation has not returned by 4-6 weeks after the operation, they are very unlikely to walk properly again. Your vet or neurologist can check for this and advise you. A few grade 5 dogs that never regain deep pain sensation eventually learn to push up to a standing position and walk a little, albeit in a wobbly way. This is called 'spinal walking', and it can be a useful way for the dog to move over short distances.

Can a dog 'recover' without learning to walk?

Some dogs go on to live a happy life without learning to walk. They get about outdoors using wheels, enjoy pushchair rides, and drag themselves around in the home.

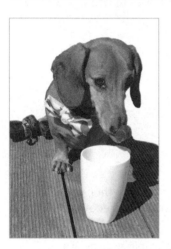

This works well for some but not all dogs and owners. Dogs that don't walk need extra home care and monitoring long term as they are also prone to skin sores and other issues. Many dogs that don't walk again are also left with poor bladder and bowel control (chapter 53). Not every owner can live with this, and it can be unsettling for some dogs as well (see Appendix 9, 'Thinking about euthanasia').

→ **See Chapter 76, 'Caring for your dog as permanently paralysed' for more information.**

BOX 11: DEEP PAIN SENSATION (DPS)

Dogs with the most severe type of IVDD (grade 5) can no longer feel their hind paws. Your vet can check for this by testing for 'deep pain sensation' if your dog cannot walk.

To test for deep pain sensation, the vet pinches a toe of a paralysed limb. If a fingertip pinch has no effect, they may try again using a tool.

A normal dog should look round and may growl or try to bite. A dog with no pain sensation might pull the leg away (this is a reflex) but appears not to notice the toe being pinched.

⚠ **IMPORTANT:** Leave the DPS test to your vet. Your recovering dog needs to be able to trust your hands.

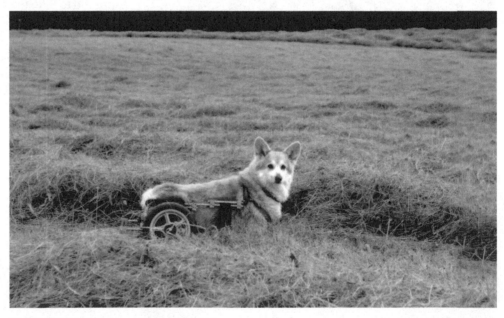

Fig 19: Many dogs get on well with wheels

My dog is not yet walking, but are they recovering?

Learning to walk is a gradual process. Be sure to give your dog enough time to do this.

Promising signs of recovery

It is unusual for a collapsed dog to just get up and walk. In the early days, watch your dog instead for more subtle signs of recovery (see box 12).

Ask your neurologist's advice if your dog does not seem to be progressing. They can assess your dog's muscle tone, reflexes and paw sensation before advising you. Your dog may need lifestyle changes (Chapter 13) and perhaps some help with physiotherapy to get them walking. Or they may just need more recovery time.

> **BOX 12: STEPPING STONES ALONG THE JOURNEY TO RECOVERY**
>
> Over days to weeks, as your dog starts to learn to walk, watch out for these signs of improvement:
>
> - Standing with a little less support from your hands.
> - Starting to stand unsupported for two or three seconds once helped into this position.
> - Twitching their leg muscles when trying to step while being sling-walked.
> - Starting to take proper steps with support from a sling.
> - Gradually starting to walk with less than full support from the sling.

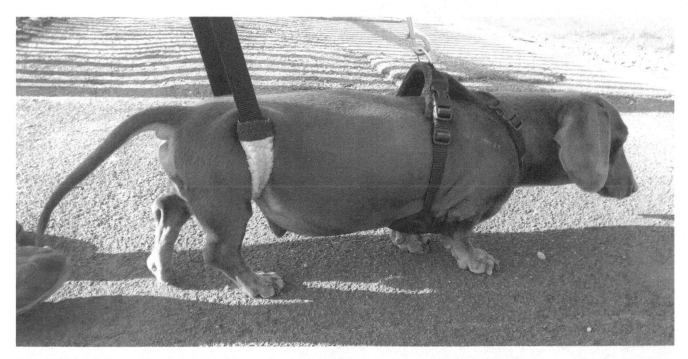

Figure 20: Starting to step with sling support is a promising sign of recovery.

SECTION 4
Your dog's recovery area

CHAPTER 16
What is crate rest and why is it needed?

Dogs act on instinct. They might rush or try to jump before their body is ready, for example if someone comes into the room, or if they are eager for their next meal.

Set up a special area to keep your dog safe. This will prevent them from hurrying across the room, getting to any slippery flooring, steps or stairs, or trying to jump on or off sofas or other furniture.

Even if your dog seems sleepy or reluctant to move on returning from the vet clinic, don't be caught out. Any dashing about could worsen their condition and land them back in hospital. Overactivity also stops inflammation from settling down.

Contain and restrain your recovering dog to keep them safe.

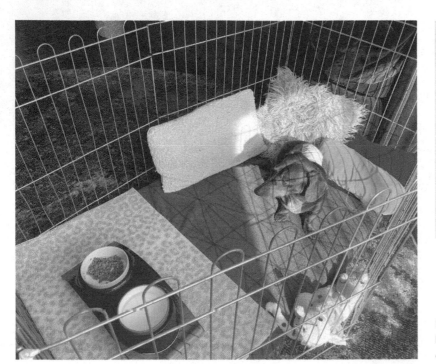

BOX 1: WHAT IS CRATE REST?

Crate rest is a period of usually several weeks or more during which your dog lives, eats, drinks and sleeps in a comfortable crate, with its door closed. Whenever your dog is outside the crate, keep them safe on a harness and lead or in your arms.

Pen rest is the same as crate rest, but uses a pen instead of a crate.

Figure 1: The crate or pen must be comfortable, secure and large enough for your dog.

CHAPTER 17
Choosing a recovery crate or pen

- 🐾 It is easier to access your dog in an open-topped pen than a crate.
- 🐾 Pens offer a larger floor area than most crates.
- 🐾 Don't use a pen if your dog might escape! Use a closed-top crate instead.

Whether to choose a pen (figure 2) or crate (figure 3) depends on your dog's size and personality. Pens are useful for larger or long-bodied dogs because they offer more floor space than crates. It's also easier to access a dog in an open-top pen than in a closed-top crate, as you can open the door and step inside. Many pens can be extended as the dog recovers, giving them more space.

However, safety is the priority! Think about how your dog usually behaves when they are healthy. Only consider using a pen if your dog will not try to escape.

If your dog is too big for a crate, but too bouncy for a high-sided pen, room rest may be the best option (chapter 25). Discuss this first with your vet.

Crates

Crates are sold as puppy crates, travel crates or recovery crates. First, check whether the crate is big enough for your dog. Your dog's travel crate or old puppy crate is probably too small.

→ **See Appendix 4 for crate sizes recommended for each breed.**

Look for a crate with a floor level exit. Most have a raised 'lip' under the door that is too high for short-limbed recovering dogs to step over. You must either lift your dog or guide them safely and slowly over the lip each time they go in and out.

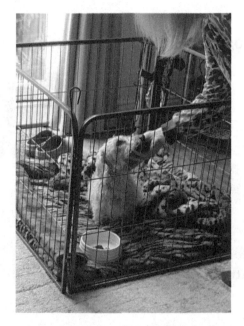

Figure 2 (left):
An open-top pen.

Figure 3 (below):
A terrier in a closed-top XXL crate.

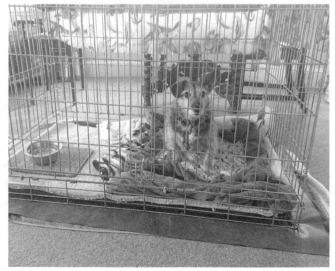

Pens

A pen should be:

✓ **Sturdy** enough to withstand some knocks and chewing. A metal structure is best.

✓ **Tall enough** so that your dog does not jump out. At least 80 cm tall is recommended, even for small dogs.

✓ **Long and wide enough** for your dog (see Chapter 18, 'Crate or pen size').

✓ **Easy for your dog to get in and out of.** If available, buy one with a floor level exit rather than a high lip. Otherwise, you will need to lift your dog over the lip, or to swing a panel open each time to let your dog in and out.

✓ **Comfortable**. It should be an inviting space for your dog.

✓ **Modular**. If the pen has panels that can be added in, this will allow you to make your dog's living space larger as they recover.

Does my dog need a crate or pen?

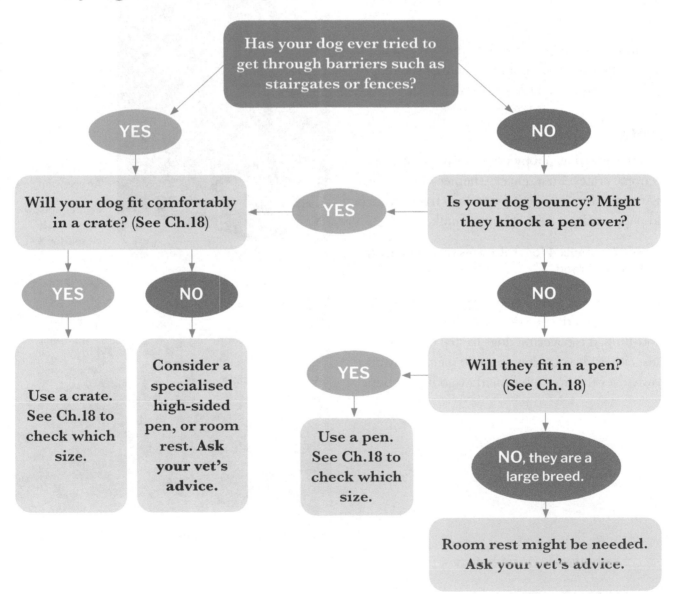

Figure 4: Flow chart, 'Does my dog need a crate or pen?'

CHAPTER 18
Crate or pen size

The right size for the crate or pen depends on the size of your dog (see Appendix 4) and on how closely they must be confined.

How closely to confine your dog: Early Rest and Late Rest

Most dogs should start with a smaller crate or pen before being moved to a larger one (see box 2).

BOX 2: EARLY REST VERSUS LATE REST

Use the smaller option, the Early Rest crate or pen:

🐾 for the first 3 weeks after injury or surgery

🐾 for first aid:

- while waiting for your first vet appointment
- or if your dog's problem has just got worse

🐾 in other situations, if advised to do so by your vet.

Check with your vet before using the larger option, the Late Rest crate or pen. This is usually used:

🐾 from 3 weeks after injury or surgery

🐾 sooner than this only if advised by your vet.

FLOOR SPACE OPTION	WHEN TO USE	WHAT'S INCLUDED
Early Rest (less space)	For the first 3 weeks after injury or surgery, for first aid, or as advised by your vet.	Bedding area, including room to eat, drink and turn around easily.
Late Rest (more space)	After 3 weeks, or as advised by your vet.	Bedding area as above, plus a standing area.

 TIP: *Think ahead to when your dog will need more space. Many pens can be extended later in recovery by adding extra panels. Crates cannot be extended. If using a crate, either get two in different sizes (perhaps borrow one and buy the other), or choose the larger size and pad the extra space with rolled blankets during Early Rest.*

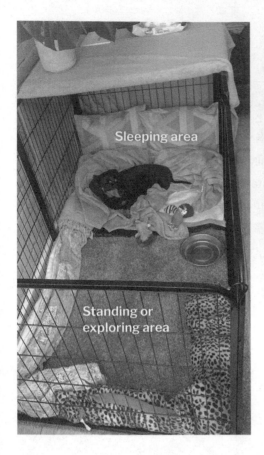

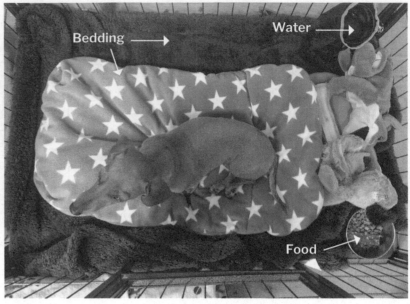

Figure 5 (above): A dachshund in an Early Rest pen. From the start of recovery, your dog needs room to stretch out comfortably and to turn around very easily. They also need space for bedding, food and water.

Figure 6 (left): A dachshund in a Late Rest pen with both a sleeping area and an area for standing or exploring.

Recommended sizes

BOX 3: RECOMMENDED CRATE AND PEN SIZES FOR FRENCH BULLDOGS AND MINIATURE DACHSHUNDS

	CRATE			PEN	
	Name	Length	Width	Square pen, length of each side	Rectangular pen
Early Rest	XL	106 cm (42 in)	70 cm (28.5 in)	70 cm to 80 cm (28 in to 32 in)	N/A
Late Rest	XXL	122 cm (48 in)	74.5 cm (29 in)	100 cm to 120 cm (39 in to 47 in)	80 cm x 160 cm (32 in x 63 in)

→ Crate and pen sizes for other breeds are listed in Appendix 4.

What pens and crates are available?

Crates

Crates are sold in standard sizes, usually labelled by their length in inches. The largest available from most outlets is about 122 cm (48 in) long and is sold as the 48 in or XXL crate.

→ **See Appendix 4 for a table of standard crate sizes.**

Don't be persuaded by the seller to buy a crate that is too small. For example, the 42 inch (XL) crate is often sold for Labradors. **During recovery, the 42 inch crate is only suitable for small dogs.** This is because they must stay in the crate for most of the day, with its door closed.

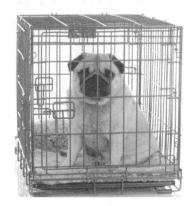

Figure 7: This medium crate is too small to use as a recovery crate for this pug.

Even the largest crates are quite narrow. They don't offer enough room for larger breeds to stretch out or to turn around, especially while recovering from a neck or back problem.

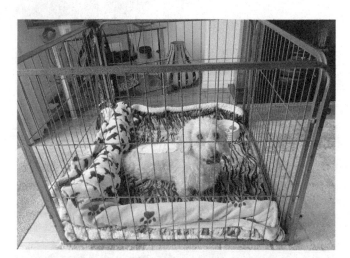

Pens

Pens come in many sizes, and some types can be made larger using extra panels.

Standard dog pens with sides 80 cm (31.5 in) high are suitable for many small dogs including most (but not all) dachshunds.

⚠ **CAUTION:** A very determined dog could escape even from a taller pen – use a crate instead.

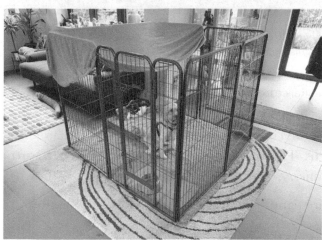

Figure 8 (top): A dog pen with sides of 80cm (31.5 inch) high and wide, used here for close confinement (Early Rest).

Figure 9 (above): Taller pens are suitable for some lively dogs. Try searching online for 'high-sided dog pen'.

CHAPTER 19
Where to put the crate or pen

Choose a position that will be practical for you and comfortable for your dog.

Which room?

If possible, put the crate or pen in a room where your dog likes to rest. It should be away from draughts and direct sunlight. Use a downstairs room if possible. Your dog will need to be helped outdoors for toileting, and stairs will be out of bounds.

 TIP: *If your confined dog seems upset by people or other dogs going past, choose a quieter spot.* Remember that they won't be able to escape from noisy family games or arguments.

Dogs have sensitive ears, so don't place the crate or pen too close to the washing machine, tumble drier, TV or other machines.

Flooring

You will either be lifting your dog in and out of their crate, or helping them to step out onto non-slip flooring. Tiles, laminate and linoleum are too slippery, so cover them with non-slip matting.

Radiators

A crate should usually be placed well away from radiators and heaters to prevent overheating. However, if your dog loves warmth and always chooses to rest by a heat source then, in a cold house, you may consider putting one short end of a pen or very large crate close to a warm radiator. A small gap between crate and radiator will prevent burns. This gives your dog a chance to rest in a warm spot. If you try this, stick to the following safety guidelines:

✓ Watch your dog very closely to start with. If they are panting, move the crate to a cooler position.

✓ Always have fresh water available inside the crate.

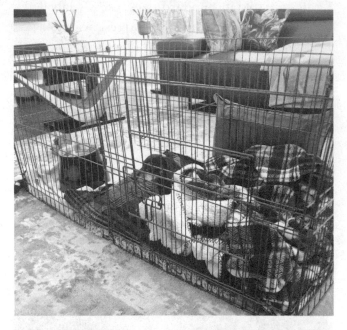

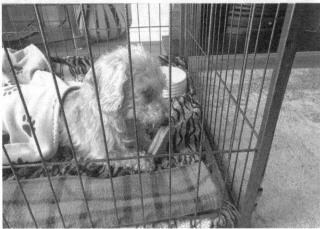

Figure 10 (top): Most dogs prefer to be in a living area that is regularly used so that they can see people coming and going.

Figure 11 (above): For safety, a rug has been placed around the entrance to this pen.

⚠ **WATCH OUT!** Flat faced dogs such as French bulldogs easily overheat. Don't put their pen or crate next to a hot radiator.

An extra crate or pen

When healthy, does your dog tend to follow you about the house? If so, you could get one or more extra crates or pens so that you can move your dog around with you during the day. Some owners have a night-time crate in their bedroom, a pen for their main living area and another pen for their home office.

A lightweight pop-up pen is a useful extra for some smaller dogs. It can be moved to any room of the house, or in good weather you could move it outdoors so that your dog can be with you if you are sitting outdoors or gardening.

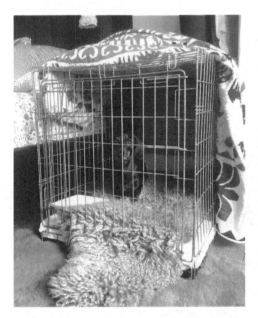

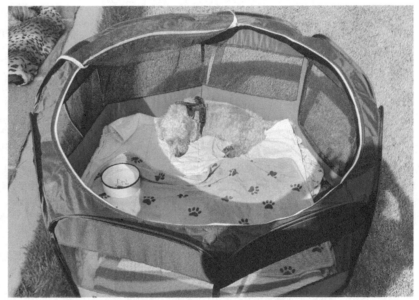

Figure 12 (above): A crate for overnight use in the bedroom.

Figure 13 (above right): A pop-up pen.

⚠ **WATCH OUT!** Only consider a pop-up pen if your dog respects barriers. They are lightweight and are for supervised use only.

CHAPTER 20

Setting up your dog's crate or pen

✓ **Cover any slick flooring** inside the crate or pen with non-slip matting.

✓ Include in the crate or pen:

- **Bedding** appropriate to your dog's needs (see chapter 22).
- **Water bowl**.
- A **food bowl** at mealtimes (or divide your dog's food ration between safe food dispensing toys).
- For incontinent dogs: vet fleece, towels or blankets and an incontinence pad.

✓ Block off any draughts.

✓ Some dogs prefer to have a sheet draped over part of the crate or pen.

During recovery, the crate or pen is your dog's own little world for most of the day and night. As well as resting, they will use this space for eating, drinking, settling down to chew on a toy, and perhaps taking some first steps. Take care to make this space comfortable.

BOX 5: THE LAYOUT OF YOUR DOG'S CRATE OR PEN DEPENDS MAINLY ON THEIR STAGE OF RECOVERY

Early Rest: Completely cover the floor area of the crate or pen with soft bedding.

Late Rest: Next to their bedding, your dog should have an area of non-slip footing where they can eat, drink, use food dispensing toys, and try to stand.

→ **See Chapter 18 for information on when to use Early Rest or Late Rest.**

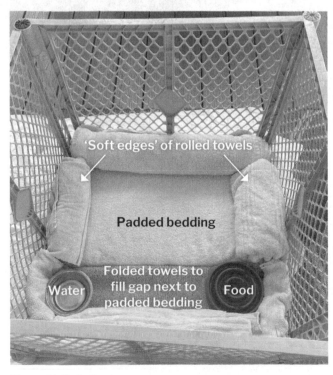

Figure 14: Early Rest pen.

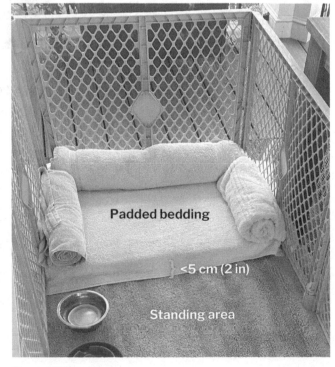

Figure 15: Late Rest pen.

How to set up the crate or pen

1. **Check what size** crate or pen to use (Chapter 18)

2. **Decide where** to put the crate or pen (Chapter 19)

3. **Consider a protective layer.** Some dogs have poor bladder control during recovery. Consider placing a sheet of plastic underneath the whole crate or pen to protect your floor. If putting a crate on carpet, place an old towel underneath so the metal does not mark the carpet.

4. **Add a non-slip layer.** Cover the floor of the pen or crate with non-slip matting if it is slippery. Any plastic sheeting must be covered with non-slip matting. See Chapter 22, 'Your dog's bedding'

5. **Add bedding** to suit your dog's needs. For Early Rest*, the bedding must cover the whole floor of the crate or pen.

6. **Add an absorbent top layer.** Place vet fleece or a blanket on top of any padded bedding. If your dog might wet the bed, put pee pads under the fleece/blanket.

7. **Add a standing area if your dog is on Late Rest*** (Chapter 21)

8. **Include a water bowl.** Clip a water bowl to the inside of the crate or pen, or tuck it into the corner where it is within easy reach but won't be knocked over.

9. **Block off any draughts** with rolled blankets or towels, or using a cot (crib) bumper.

10. **Cover part of it.** If your dog likes to be cosy, cover part of the crate or pen with a sheet.

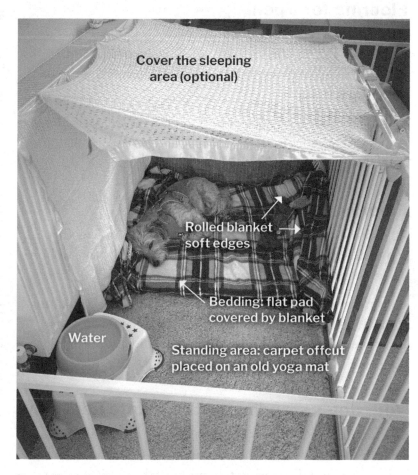

Cover the sleeping area (optional)

Rolled blanket soft edges

Bedding: flat pad covered by blanket

Water

Standing area: carpet offcut placed on an old yoga mat

Figure 16: A Late Rest pen for a dog that can walk.

*For guidance on Late and Early rest, see Chapter 18, 'Crate or pen size'.

CHAPTER 21

The flooring and standing area in the crate or pen

SUMMARY

Put a non-slip base layer in the crate or pen to:

❁ prevent bedding from sliding around.

❁ make it safer and easier for your dog to stand and walk.

Flooring for a pen

The floor of your room forms the base for most styles of dog pen. Place the pen on carpet if possible. Non-slip footing helps your dog recover, and a grippy surface makes the pen more stable.

If using a room with a slippery floor, put down a rug or non-slip matting and set the pen on this. Put your dog's bedding directly onto this base layer.

Flooring for a crate

Check your crate before you set it up. Many come with a removable plastic base. Remove this base if it is very wobbly. Your dog needs a stable base of support.

Cover the entire floor inside the crate with non-slip matting. Your dog's bedding goes on top of this. The non-slip base layer prevents bedding from sliding around and is safer for your dog to stand and walk on.

Your dog's standing area: for Late Rest only

During Late Rest*, your dog should have a standing area next to their bedding. They can use this space to eat and drink, use food dispensing toys and watch people coming and going from a different angle.

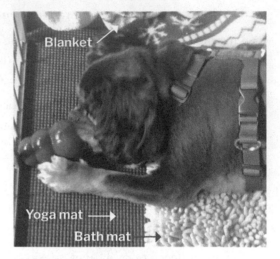

Blanket

Yoga mat →

Bath mat →

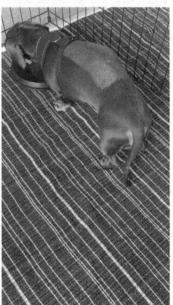

Figure 17 (above): Yoga matting is used as the base layer for this pen.

Figure 18 (left): This pen is placed on a non-slip rug. This is a good surface on which to learn to walk.

The standing area must have good non-slip footing.

Options include:

✓ **Vet fleece.** The rubber-backed version can be placed directly on slick flooring. Standard fleece must instead be placed on carpet or non-slip matting so that it doesn't slide about when stepped on.

✓ **Rubber-backed fluffy bathmats** (figure 17) can be used instead of vet fleece

✓ **Carpet or rug** if the dog's pen has been placed on this

✓ **Rubber matting**, e.g. yoga matting.

⚠ **WATCH OUT!** Some dogs will try to chew anything that is put in their crate or pen.

*For guidance on Late and Early rest, see Chapter 18, 'Crate or pen size'.

CHAPTER 22
Your dog's bedding

Bedding during Early Rest and Late Rest

During Early Rest, the bedding should fill the crate or pen. Fill any gaps between the bed and the edge of the crate or pen with rolled blankets or towels. This will prevent your dog from rolling down into a gap or getting a leg stuck.

During Late Rest, make it easy and safe for your dog to reach their standing area. Check that the bedding is:

✓ easy to access – avoid beds that have a raised front edge

✓ thin enough for your dog to get on and off very easily.

For safe access, bedding should be no more than 5 cm (2 in) thick for a small dog, and no more than 10 cm (4 in) thick for larger breeds.

→ **See Chapter 18, 'Crate or pen size' for a note on when to use Early Rest or Late Rest.**

Layered bedding

Most dogs need some padding. This goes under a top layer such as blanket or fleece.

Standard padding

Use a flat rectangular or oval pad that is large enough for your dog to stretch out on fully. Good options include:

• your dog's usual bed or its pad insert

• a crate mat or crate pad

• a folded blanket.

💡 *If there is a gap between the edges of the crate and the foam pad, fill it carefully by tucking in towels or blankets.*

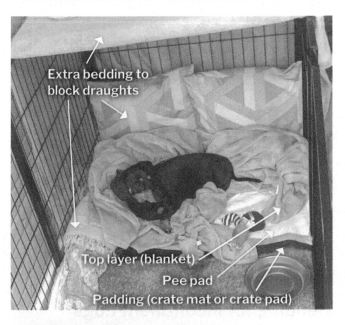

KEY POINTS

🐾 Choose a bed that is large enough for your dog to stretch out on comfortably.

🐾 Your dog should rest on a top layer of fleece, towelling or blanket.

🐾 Most dogs need padding. This goes under the top layer.

Extra bedding to block draughts

Top layer (blanket)

Pee pad

Padding (crate mat or crate pad)

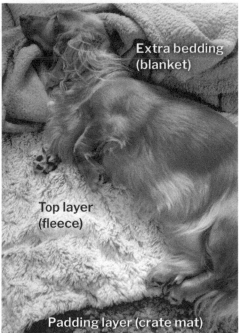

Extra bedding (blanket)

Top layer (fleece)

Padding layer (crate mat)

Figure 19 (above): The sleeping area of a Late Rest pen, showing the layers of bedding.

Figure 20 (left): Bedding layers.

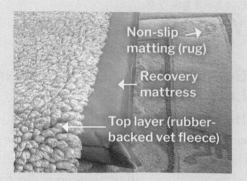

BOX 6: SPECIALISED PADDING

ASK YOUR VET. Thicker padding is only needed for a few dogs with IVDD, usually heavier breeds or those that cannot prop themselves up or change position. Your vet can advise you.

If needed, use a purpose-made recovery mattress, or ask a foam supplier to cut a block of memory foam to fit the base of the crate or pen and to cover it for you.

 WATCH OUT! Some recovery mattresses are too thick for dogs to get on and off easily. They're best reserved for collapsed dogs that are not trying to move much.

Figure 21: A recovery mattress for a large breed on room rest.

The top layer of bedding

Put a soft, washable layer on top of the padding. Use one of the following:

- ✓ a machine-washable blanket
- ✓ vet fleece*
- ✓ a towel

Shallow bedding – no padding

A few dogs are comfortable with no padding, especially if they have always preferred to sleep on the floor rather than on a bed. Padding is not essential if your dog can walk, get up and change position without your help.

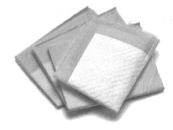

Figure 22: For shallow bedding, simply provide one or two layers of blanket or vet fleece*

Bedding for incontinent dogs

Some IVDD dogs may pee or poo without realising it, either where they lay or on rising. If your dog has poor bladder or bowel control, use absorbent washable surfaces such as vet fleece*, blankets or towelling as a top layer throughout the crate or pen and keep spares to hand in case of soiling.

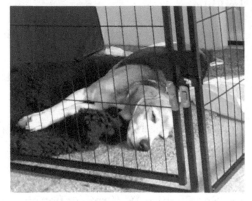

Figure 23: Incontinence pads (pee pads).

Pee pads

Place pee pads just under your dog's fleece or blanket to catch any run-through.

Layering pee pads and bedding

- Pee pads can be scratchy against the dog's skin, so the soft bedding layer is best put on top (see figure 19).
- Some owners find it more practical to put the pee pads on top of the bedding, directly under the dog. This might not be quite as comfortable, but could make your life easier by reducing the amount of washing needed, especially if your dog keeps peeing little and often.

⚠ **IMPORTANT:** Check the bedding and pee pads frequently and change them whenever they are wet or soiled.

Vet fleece is best avoided for unneutered male dogs as it may irritate delicate skin.

Optional: Protective underlayer

A plastic sheet underneath your dog's crate or pen will protect the floor. You could also wrap their pad or mattress in a plastic bin liner if it is not waterproof. Cover any plastic with bedding and/or washable non-slip matting. Plastic is too slippery for a recovering dog to try and move about on.

Extra bedding

💡 **TOP TIP:** *Check for draughts down by the floor at dog level, particularly at night.*

Stop any draughts using:

* a bolster cushion (figure 24)
* a blanket tucked between the wall and the crate
* rolled towels around the edges of the crate (figure 14)
* or a cot (crib) bumper wrapped around the crate.

Covering part of the crate or pen with a sheet or blanket may also help your dog to settle down (see figure 19). Keep at least one side of the crate uncovered to allow for some airflow, and so that you can check on them.

If your dog usually sleeps covered

Include a favourite blanket or old towel if your dog loves to snuggle down. Keep an eye on them and be sure that they don't get stuck.

Include an old favourite

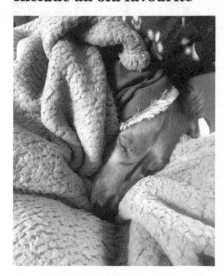
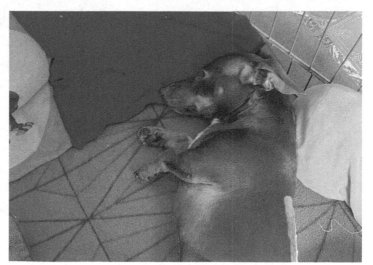

Figures 25 & 26: Include items that smell familiar to your dog if possible, such as their own towel, a favourite toy, or a small cushion that they have always liked to rest against.

BOX 7: BEST AVOIDED: A TOILET ZONE IN THE PEN

Some owners choose to cover part of the crate or pen floor with either newspaper or incontinence pads in case their dog needs to pee unexpectedly. This is best avoided as they are slippery and make poor surfaces for dogs that are learning to walk.

If you must put a toilet zone in the pen (perhaps your dog had previously been trained to pee on paper), make it safer by placing non-slip mats directly under the paper or pads.

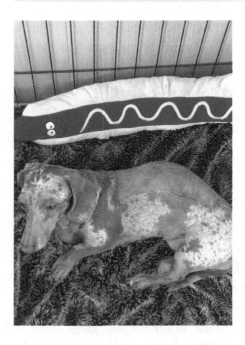

Figure 24: A bolster cushion to block draughts.

CHAPTER 23

Introducing your dog to the recovery space

Make your dog's first experience of the crate or pen a pleasant one. This will help them accept it as a positive place: their own comfortable recovery hideout.

Before your dog sees the crate or pen

Before your dog first enters the crate, set it up with comfortable bedding, a draught-free place to rest, food, water and their favourite toys. Check that the floor of the crate offers good footing and does not wobble, otherwise your dog will lose confidence as soon as they try to move.

Dogs are quick to pick up on our emotions, so do your best to keep your voice positive and kind when introducing them to their recovery space.

When your dog enters the crate or pen

Have food ready inside the crate when your dog first sees it. This could be a meal in a bowl, or part of your dog's usual food ration divided between food dispensing toys. Lick mats and snuffle mats are useful for keeping dogs absorbed during early IVDD recovery. Once your dog is focused on eating, close the crate door gently and step away quietly.

TOP TIPS

✓ Make the crate or pen comfortable before showing it to your dog.

✓ Handle your dog gently and keep your voice kind and positive.

✓ Offer food in the crate or pen. Either feed this from a bowl or divide the daily ration between food dispensing toys.

✓ While the dog is focused on eating, close the crate door gently.

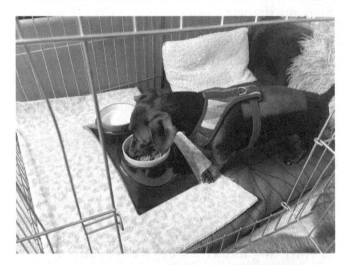

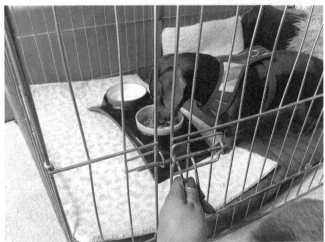

Fig 27a (top): When your dog first sees the crate or pen, have food in there ready for them.

Fig 27b (above): Close the door quietly once your dog is focused on eating.

CHAPTER 24
Safety outside the crate or pen

Why take special care?

Dogs act on instinct, sometimes rushing or trying to jump even if part of their body is paralysed. This could happen if the doorbell rings, mail arrives, or for no apparent reason at all. Don't be caught out. These dogs can move surprisingly fast when we least expect it, and this could cause permanent damage.

SUMMARY

Keep your dog safe whenever they are outside the crate or pen. They could be:

✓ in your arms.

✓ on harness and lead.

✓ safely secured in a dog stroller, with close supervision.

✓ by your side with your hand holding their harness.

When to keep dogs safe

The crate or pen is a handy tool if used well. While your dog is shut inside, they cannot run, jump or access stairs, other dogs, balls or slick flooring. However, there are times such as outdoor toilet breaks and vet appointments when your dog must be brought out of this space. You may also need to bring them out for other reasons, such as for exercises or massage, perhaps to sit together now and again, and eventually to start short lead-walks.

Avoid all slick flooring. Lift your dog over it or put down non-slip mats.

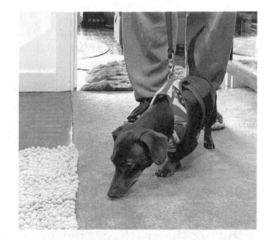

Leaving the crate

Don't let your dog push past you as you open the crate or pen door. It's useful to leave them wearing a well-fitting harness (see Chapter 26 'Your dog's harness'). As you open the crate door, put your hand on the top strap of the harness. This stops them slipping out past you, and gives you time to attach a lead or to lift and carry them.

Some crates and pens have a high lip at their exit. If so, do one of the following:

- Lift your dog over the lip
- Open the pen by swinging a panel open so that your dog can walk out at floor level.

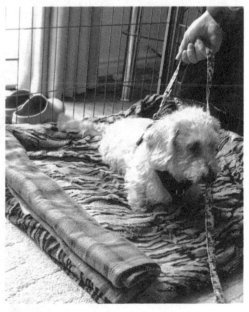

Figure 28 (top): A dog safely restrained on a lead. Non-slip matting makes it easier for dogs to walk.

Figure 29 (above): This dog leaves the pen on the lead. Two pen panels have been swung open for easy access.

Getting from crate to garden

If your dog is small enough, expect to do a lot of lifting and carrying. At toilet break time, lift them from the crate or pen, and carry over any slick flooring, floor level changes, stairs and doorsteps, to access a safe area of grass outdoors. (See Chapter 31, 'Carrying your dog')

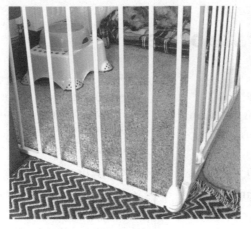

Figure 30: Make it safer for your dog to step out by placing a rug or non-slip matting just outside the crate or pen if your floor is slick.

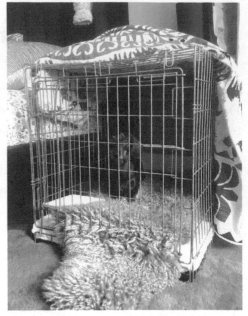

Dogs that are too large to lift must be guided through the home carefully on harness and lead, using a sling if needed for extra support. First create a safe route. If you have slick flooring, lay a pathway of non-slip runners from the pen to the garden door. Plan how to get your dog over your doorstep before you start. Depending on your dog's size and ability, you may need to lift them over the step or have them step over it very slowly on harness and lead with sling support.

During the crate rest period, don't let your dog wander loose in the room or garden.

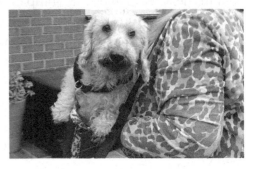

Figure 31 (top): A sheepskin draped over the metal crate lip makes it easier for a dog to step out. It also doubles as a bedding top layer.

Figure 32 (above): Carry your dog over the garden step.

Figure 33 (left): Always keep hold of your dog's harness if you place them on a sofa or bed.

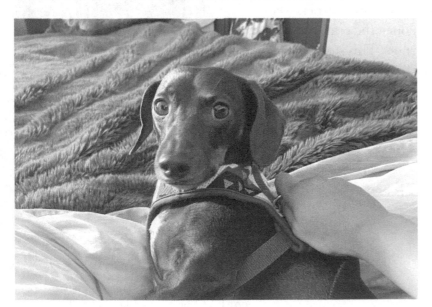

⚠ **WATCH OUT!** Never leave your recovering dog on a raised surface. Dogs with IVDD are at high risk of falls.

CHAPTER 25
Room rest

What is room rest?

During room rest the dog recovers in a room with the door closed instead of in a crate or pen. They stay in this room for all activities except for outdoor toilet breaks and other essentials such as clinic appointments. When outside the room, keep your dog on a lead (with sling support if needed), or in your arms, or safely constrained and supervised in a dog stroller.

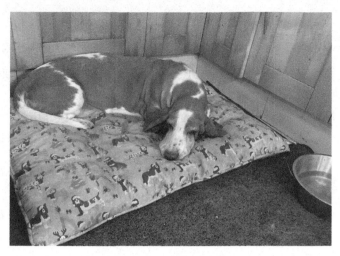

Figure 34: Room rest is sometimes used for larger breeds.

When to use room rest

For dogs with IVDD, room rest should only be used in a few exceptional cases and only after discussion with your vet.

Crate or pen rest is generally much safer. In a crate or pen, the dog cannot jump on furniture, drag across the room to greet you, or slip out of the room if someone opens the door.

> ⚠ **CAUTION:** Check with your vet before using room rest. Crate or pen rest is safer for most IVDD dogs.

The main reason to use room rest is

...if the dog is too large for any crate, but too bouncy to stay within an open-topped pen.

SAFETY ADVICE

Avoid room rest if:

- ✗ someone might open the door carelessly.
- ✗ your rooms are large or open plan.
- ✗ flooring is slick.
- ✗ your dog might try to jump on furniture in this room.
- ✗ other dogs will be coming in and out of the room.

Choosing a room

A quiet, familiar place

Your dog will recover better if you choose a room in which they are already used to relaxing. Most dogs expect regular interaction with their owner, so consider a small living space or study where you spend much of your time. Avoid through-rooms or hallways: it's hard for dogs to settle down if people keep opening doors and moving past.

TOP TIPS

Choosing a recovery room

- ✓ Choose a small room that is familiar to your dog.
- ✓ Avoid furniture if your dog might jump on it.
- ✓ Avoid any steps. Flooring must be on one level.
- ✓ Choose a room with a door that can be kept shut to prevent escape.
- ✗ Avoid slick flooring. If flooring is slick, cover it with non-slip matting.

Setting the room up

Set the room up comfortably for recovery, including the following:

✓ Non-slip flooring. Put mats down if the floor is slippery.

✓ Water bowl within easy reach.

✓ Bedding (see Chapter 22, 'Your dog's bedding').

✓ Food either in a bowl or in safe food-dispensing toys (see Chapter 35, 'Toys').

Include items that smell familiar to your dog if possible, such as their own towel or a favourite blanket or soft toy.

Your dog should eat in their recovery room. Either feed them from their bowl, or divide their usual food ration between safe food-dispensing toys and offer these at intervals during the day.

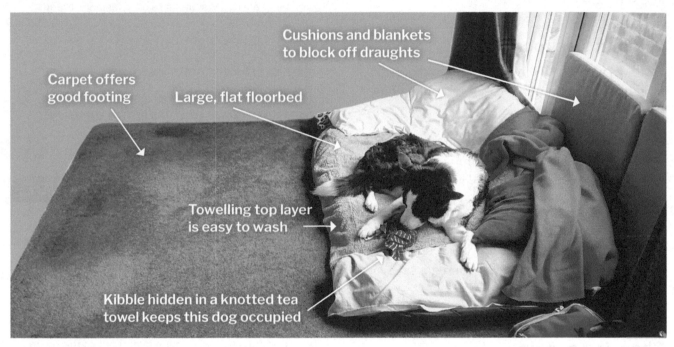

Figure 36: Provide a good floor bed during room rest.

Bedding

During room rest, your dog's bed must be:

✓ Large enough for them to lie on when fully stretched out.

✓ Easy for them to access. Avoid beds:

• that are raised off the floor

• with a raised front edge

Check for draughts around where your dog rests. Tuck rolled blankets behind the bedding to block these out if needed.

→ Go to... For more details, see Chapter 22, 'Your dog's bedding'.

Flooring

Flooring must be non-slip during recovery from IVDD. Laminate, wooden, tiled or vinyl floors are too slippery. Choose a carpeted room if possible. Otherwise cover any slick flooring with non-slip matting.

Non-slip matting

Rubber backed rugs or runners can be bought online or from homeware or some hardware stores. Rubber mat tiles designed for children's play areas are also suitable. Door mats, old yoga matting and rubber-backed bathmats can be used if needed to fill any gaps.

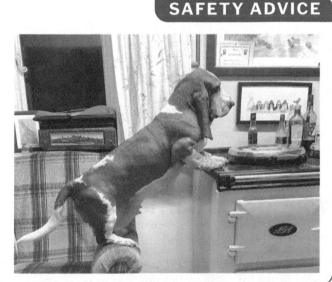

SAFETY ADVICE

Safety considerations

The recovery room must be on one level. It should have step-free access to the outdoor toilet area. otherwise you will have to lift your dog in and out. Good footing is essential, so choose a carpeted room if possible.

 AVOID THIS. One of the main challenges of room rest is preventing the dog from jumping onto furniture, so avoid or remove any armchairs, beds, sofas etc.

Figure 35: Don't get caught out: dogs sometimes surprise us in what they try to do.

SECTION 5
Basic skills and equipment for recovery

This section covers the most essential skills and equipment needed for recovery.

Basic equipment:

Chapter 26: Your dog's harness

Chapter 27: Your dog's lead

Chapter 28: Hindquarter slings

Using this equipment:

Chapter 29: Using the lead

Chapter 30: Using the sling

Other basic skills:

Chapter 31: Carrying your dog

Chapter 32: 'Together time' – sitting safely with your dog

Chapter 33: Caring for your dog's surgical wound

CHAPTER 26
Your dog's harness

A good harness fits around the chest, supporting and restraining your dog around their centre of gravity. It's one of the most useful tools in helping a dog recover.

Choosing a harness

A good harness

Harnesses come in many shapes and types. For your dog's recovery, choose one that fits quite snugly and allows their front legs to move freely.

Look for a harness with:

✓ A Y-shaped front (see figure 1)

✓ The lead attachment on the top (see figure 2)

The harness should be

- Easy to adjust. The best harnesses have adjustable straps around the chest, neck and between the front legs.

- Easy to take on and off

    ✓ Harnesses with a clip on each side of the chest are usually easiest.

    ✓ If your dog is wearing an Elizabethan collar, or if they dislike having their head or neck touched, choose a design with a neck clip so you don't have to slide anything over their head.

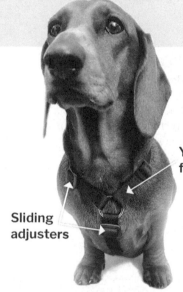

Y-shaped front

Sliding adjusters

Figure 1: Choose a harness with a Y-shaped front.

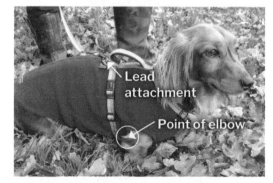

Lead attachment

Point of elbow

Figure 2: The lead should attach to a D-ring on the top of the harness, just behind the level of the point of the elbow.

Choose a harness that is comfortable enough to leave on your dog for most of the day at home. Some dogs are particular about the feel of the fabric on their skin. They may show a strong preference for one type of harness. Consider trying out a couple of types to find the best long-term solution.

Harnesses that are best avoided during recovery

Avoid:

- ✗ A harness with a slider or noose that tightens over the dog's back or neck if they pull on the lead. These are sometimes sold as 'no pull' harnesses.
- ✗ A horizontal strap across the front of the body. This will press either on the neck or shoulders (figure 5).
- ✗ A 'step-in' harness with an upside-down V shape over each elbow (figure 6) as this could restrict the front legs.
- ✗ A harness made of very stretchy fabric, as this may not give enough support.

BOX 1. HARNESSES FOR VARIOUS DOG BREEDS

For small breeds, including miniature dachshunds and French bulldogs, use an adjustable harness with webbing, neoprene or fleecy straps, or consider a fabric vest-style harness.

For greyhounds and lurchers, use a harness with strong fleecy straps. It should adjust to fit their narrow, deep-chested body, and allow extra adjustment to fit a jacket underneath in cold weather.

For large breeds and dogs that pull on the lead, a sturdy non-stretchy design is essential. It could be made of webbing or tough neoprene. For taller dogs that cannot yet use their hind limbs, the Help 'Em Up harness is recommended (see figure 3). This includes two sections: a front chest harness and a rear lift component.

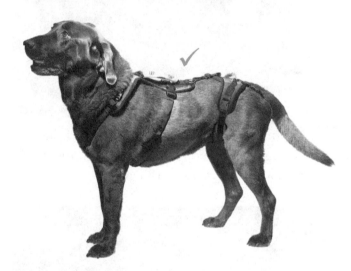

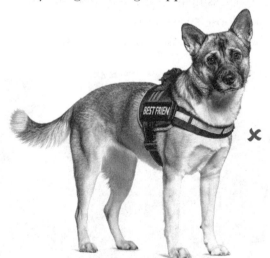

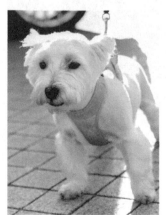

Figure 3 (top right): The Help 'Em Up harness is a good harness and sling combination for large breeds.

Figure 4 (bottom right): A vest style harness with a good Y-shaped front. Some vest harnesses are made of fabric that is too stretchy. Check before buying.

Figure 5 (top left): A horizontal strap across the chest is best avoided.

Figure 6 (bottom left): Avoid an upside-down V over the elbows.

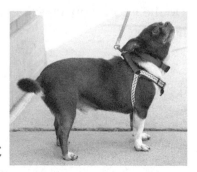

Getting the harness on

If your dog has never worn a harness, help them get used to the idea by making their first experience of it positive.

The pictures show a small Mekuti harness being fitted on a standard dachshund. This design goes over the dog's head before being fastened.

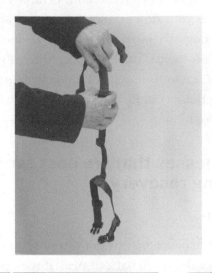

1. Before you start

Loosen the straps before fitting the harness for the first time.

Hold the harness up to check which way round it goes. The clip for the lead should be on top.

2. Putting the harness on:

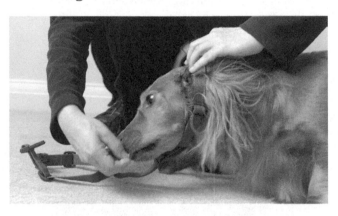

For designs that go on over the dog's head, start by offering a small food reward through the head hole to boost your dog's confidence.

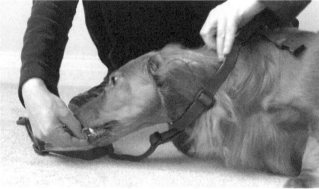

Slide the harness neatly over your dog's head, holding any loose straps or buckles out of the way so that they don't knock and startle your dog.

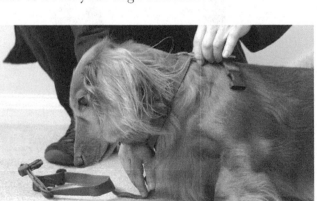

Pass the remaining straps between your dog's front legs.

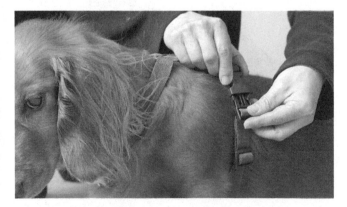

Do the harness up, checking that the straps are not twisted.

3. Adjusting the harness:

Loosen or tighten each strap as needed. The fit should be quite snug all the way around so that you can fit just one finger width easily under each strap (see pictures below). Check that the harness does not pinch anywhere around the shoulders or elbows.

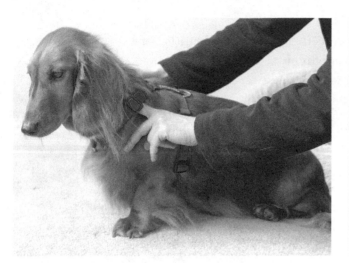 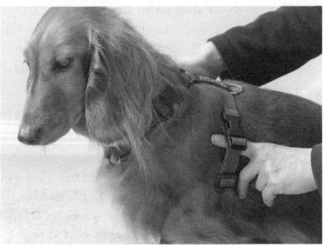

TIP: *Keep your dog's confidence up by talking to them as you adjust the harness.*

BOX 2: WHY USE A HARNESS?

❧ **For safety outdoors.** Slow your dog and keep them safe using a lead attached to the harness instead of pulling on their neck. The neck includes part of their spine and contains other delicate structures.

❧ **For safety indoors.** The top of the harness acts as a safety 'grab handle'. Use this to steady your dog or stop them from rushing off.

❧ **To improve weight distribution.** The lead attaches to the harness close to the dog's centre of gravity, helping to spread their body weight safely and evenly between all four limbs.

❧ **To encourage calmness and confidence.** If your dog is feeling unsettled, restless or sore, or is struggling to balance, then something tightening around their neck may cause them to panic. Using a harness helps them balance more calmly.

❧ **To allow natural behaviours.** A harness gives your dog freedom to move their head and neck as they wish, even when restrained on a short lead. This allows them to look about, sniff the air and sniff the ground without losing their balance.

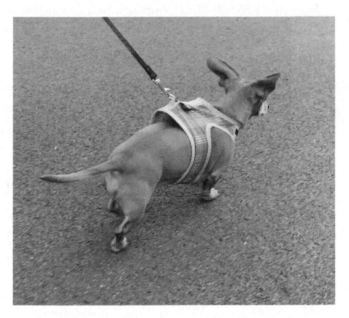

Figure 8: Harness and lead provide reassurance and support, like a tightrope walker's balancing pole.

CHAPTER 27
Your dog's lead

A lead is essential during recovery because

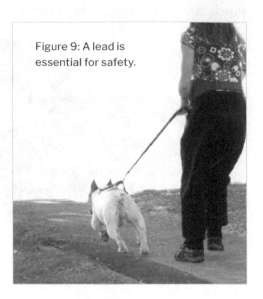

Figure 9: A lead is essential for safety.

* **It keeps your dog safe:** Dogs act on instinct. They might lurch forward, leap about or even try to run off on seeing a pigeon, squirrel, or cat, or in some cases for no apparent reason. Don't be caught out. Uncontrolled activity can cause further damage to the spine.

* **It slows their front end,** so that their hind legs have a chance to step. This will help your dog learn to walk normally again.

Use your dog's lead for all their outdoor toilet breaks. You may also find it helpful to use the lead indoors at times.

Don't let your dog go off the lead until the vet or surgeon says it's safe.

Choosing a lead

A lead that provides fine control is best during recovery. If you don't yet have an ideal lead, start with what you have before buying a new one.

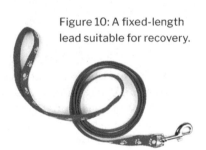

Figure 10: A fixed-length lead suitable for recovery.

During recovery, the lead should be:

✓ fixed length (not extendable).

✓ a design with a clip, to attach it to your dog's harness.

✓ comfortable to hold. Nylon, fleece or very soft leather are suitable.

Avoid:

✗ extendable leads. Their large unwieldy handle doesn't allow fine control even if the lead is set at a short length.

✗ slip leads, choke chains, and anything else that could tighten around your dog's neck.

✗ leads with a stretchy, elastic or bungee section, because they offer less support.

BOX 3: LEAD LENGTH

You may need two leads, a shorter one for sling-walking, and a longer lead once your dog can walk without a sling. Choose a slightly longer lead if you are tall or if your dog is low to the ground.

Suggested lead length:

* **For sling-walking a small breed,** around 70 to 100 cm (28 to 39 inches).

* **Once your dog can walk without a sling**

  * For use with two hands (the recommended, safest option) – 160 to 200 cm (63 to 79 inches).

  * For use with one hand (for example, if you have an injured arm) – 60 to 75 cm (24 to 30 inches).

 TIP: *If unsure which length to buy, choose a longer lead, and gather any excess up in your hand.*

CHAPTER 28
Hindquarter slings

If your dog cannot walk without falling, use a sling to support their hindquarters (see Chapter 30, 'Using the sling'). It's best not to use a sling if your dog can already walk unsupported. Otherwise, they may start to rely on it for support.

Choosing a sling

There are two main types of hindquarter sling. Some loop under the belly, while others fit around the hind legs.

A sling looped under the belly

This is a simple option, particularly useful for smaller breeds. Choose one lined with sheepskin or other soft fabric. It should have handles that can be adjusted to suit your height so that you don't need to stoop.

> **BOX 4: IMPROVISING A SLING**
>
> In an emergency, make do with:
>
> - a long towel for large dogs.
> - a scarf for medium breeds and standard dachshunds (see figure 12).
> - a fluffy bathrobe belt for miniature dachshunds and other very small dogs.

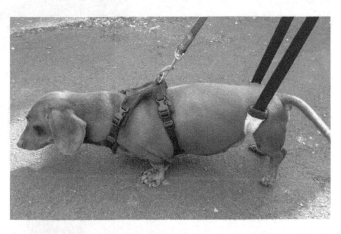

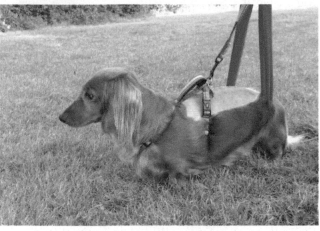

Figure 11 (top): A sling that loops under the belly is suitable for smaller breeds such as dachshunds and French bulldogs.

Figure 12 (above): A scarf used as a sling for a standard dachshund.

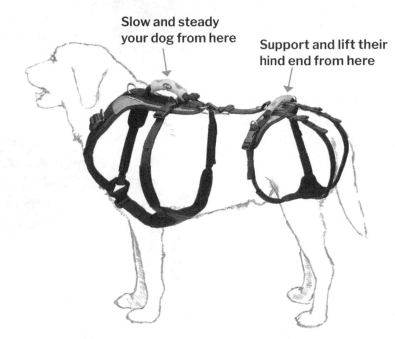

Slow and steady your dog from here

Support and lift their hind end from here

Figure 13: The Help 'Em Up harness is a hard-wearing adjustable sling, particularly useful for heavy dogs and larger breeds. It's made of a chest harness that attaches to a 'hip lift'.

A sling that fits around the hind legs

Slings that fit around the hind legs (see figures 13 and 14) are recommended for heavier dogs and for those that are very weak. They can be quite fiddly to put on and take off but, once fitted, they do a great job at supporting the dog's weight.

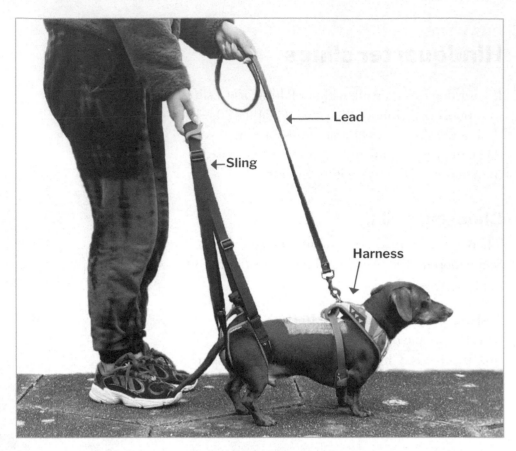

Lead

←**Sling**

Harness

Figure 14:
Hip lift slings with long handles can be used for smaller breeds.

A sling for use with one hand

It is usually best to hold the sling handle(s) in one hand, and your dog's lead in the other hand. This allows the sling and lead to act in different directions. The lead slows your dog down, while the sling provides uplift to prevent falls.

If you can only use one hand to assist your dog, use a sling that connects to their harness lead. You won't have such fine control over their balance, but it will stop them from falling.

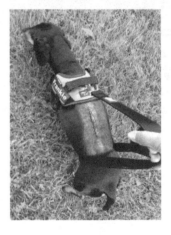

Figure 15 (left):
The Gingerlead sling can be used with one hand.

Figure 16 (below): Folding a wider sling in half for a male dog.

A sling for male dogs

If the sling comes too far forward then it will stop a male dog from peeing. Choose a narrow sling to go under his belly as in figure 11, or a hip lift sling as in figure 14.

 TIP: *As a temporary solution, you can fold a wider sling back on itself to give him room to pee.*

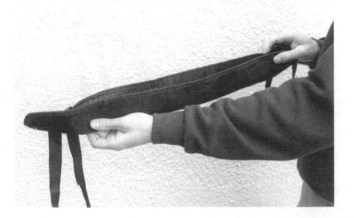

CHAPTER 29
Using the lead

Use the lead with good technique to help your dog learn to walk properly.

How to hold the lead

Two-handed lead hold

Holding the lead with two hands will give you better control so is strongly recommended.

Figure 17 and 18: Holding the lead with two hands.

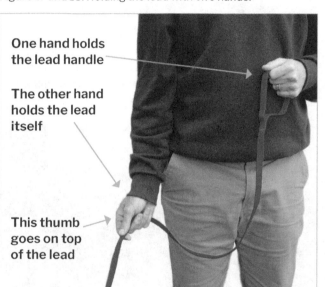

One hand holds the lead handle

The other hand holds the lead itself

This thumb goes on top of the lead

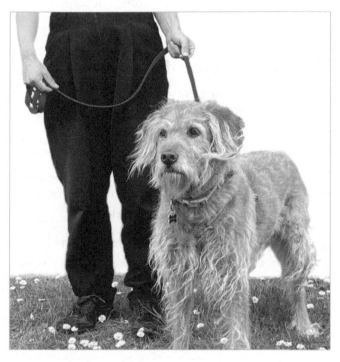

One-handed lead hold

There may be moments when you only have one hand free to hold your dog's lead. Gather up any excess lead in your hand so that the lead is just about taut. It should not hang in a loop.

Place your thumb on top of the lead loops if you can. For best control, your thumb should point along the top of the lead towards your dog.

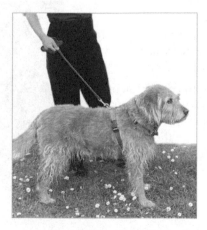

Figure 19: Holding the lead with one hand.

BOX 5: USING A LEAD DURING SLING WALKING

If your dog cannot walk unaided, support them with a sling. Hold the lead in one hand, and the sling in the other. Gather up any excess lead in your hand.

→ See chapter 30, 'Using the sling'.

How to position yourself

Allow your dog to walk and stand a little ahead of you whenever they are on the lead. This will help them to use their hind paws properly and safely. Your hand should always be behind the lead clip.

Walk on your dog's weaker side if they have one. For example, if they tend to knuckle, drag or scuff their right hind paw, then walk on their right side (see figure 20). If your dog's hind legs are equally strong, then spend half the time walking on each side.

How to slow your dog

Many dogs are enthusiastic and try to hurry ahead before their body is ready for this. Whenever your dog rushes forward, use the lead to slow them. They should be walking, not trotting, during early recovery. This will feel much slower than you are used to moving, especially if your dog is a small or short-legged breed.

To your dog, slow, careful walking may feel like a challenge. They may find it easier at first to rush along, taking chaotic steps and dragging or crossing their paws. Use thumb tip or fingertip pressure on the lead to slow your dog down when needed (see box 6).

SUMMARY

✓ Stay level with your dog's tail or a little behind this.

✓ Keep the lead pointing back from its clip.

✓ Walk on your dog's weaker side, if they have one.

✗ Don't get ahead of your dog: if your dog stops, then so should you.

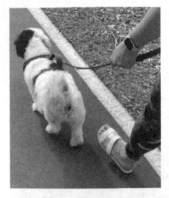

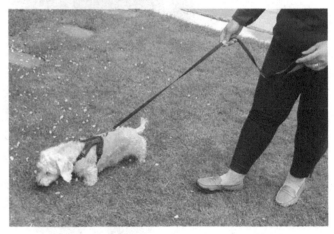

Figure 20 (left): This owner is correctly positioned just behind her dog and to one side.

Figure 21 (below): Slow your dog's front end to give their hind paws a better chance to step.

Remember...Your dog needs to learn to walk slowly properly before going faster.

BOX 6: FINE CONTROL OF THE LEAD

Lead tension. The part of the lead between your hand and the dog's harness should not hang in a loop. Instead, keep the lead just about taut, so you have some control 'just in case'.

A give-take action on the lead. With your thumb on top of the lead, you will feel when your dog lurches forward or starts to hurry ahead. Use fingertip pressure on the lead to slow your dog for a moment when needed. Then release the pressure a little so they can travel forward.

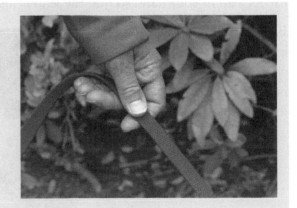

What to do if your dog gets over-excited

Dogs sometimes get excited and try to rush forward, for example if they see a bird or cat. If this happens when your dog is on the lead then don't worry, their chest harness will steady them safely. Just remember to:

- ✓ keep two hands on the lead
- ✓ stay next to or just behind your dog's hindquarters
- ✓ keep calm.

If your dog turns to face the other way, turn with them. Reposition your feet so that you remain just behind and to one side of them.

Encouraging your dog to move forward

Be patient. Your recovering dog might find it hard to walk at times, and they may be too weak or tired to go any faster.

> **Never pull your dog forward from the lead, even if they are dawdling.**

Pulling your dog forward from the lead prompts them to tip their bodyweight forward onto their front paws. This would lead to an unhelpful coordination pattern, in which they do not use their hind legs properly but lean instead on their front legs.

How to start moving

Encourage your dog to move by facing the way that you want to go and talking to them, e.g. "Come on, Jack!". You can also point forward with the handle end of the lead to prompt your dog to start walking if needed.

TOP TIPS

Even when you want your dog to go faster, keep the main part of the lead pointing back from its clip.

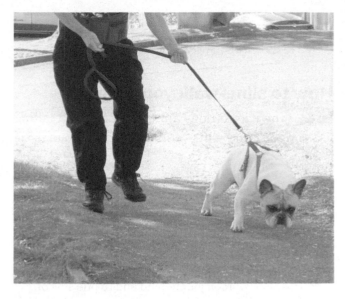

Figure 22: If your dog gets overexcited, stay calm and keep two hands on their lead.

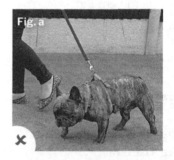 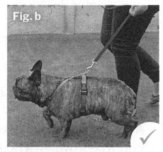

Figure 23: Don't pull your dog forward from the lead (fig. a). Keep the lead pointing back from its clip (fig. b).

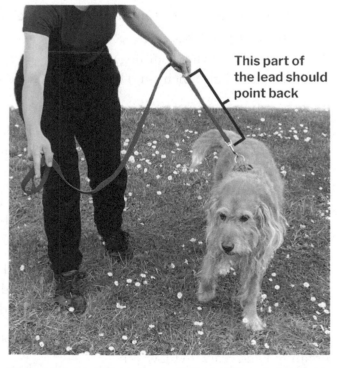

This part of the lead should point back

Figure 24: Point straight ahead with the handle end of the lead if you want your dog to move forward.

CHAPTER 30
Using the sling

How to sling-walk your dog

Use a sling if your dog cannot walk without falling. Once stronger and more stable, they'll need less and less support, and will eventually be able to make a gradual transition to walking without one.

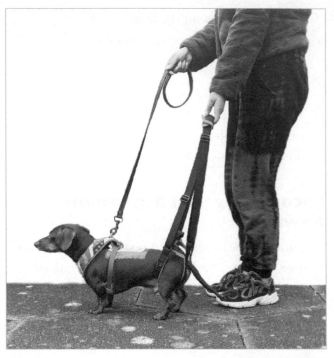

> **TOP TIPS**
>
> **BOX 7: USING THE SLING**
>
> ✓ Have your dog on harness and lead during sling-walking.
>
> ✓ Hold the lead in one hand, and the sling in the other hand.
>
> ✓ Position yourself just behind and to one side of your dog's tail.
>
> ✓ Lift the sling just enough so that your dog's hind paws do not drag along the ground.
>
> ✓ Walk slowly, using the lead as brakes if your dog tries to rush ahead.

Using the lead and sling at the same time

Always have your dog on the lead when you are sling-walking them.

This will improve their:

* ❧ **safety.** The lead stops your dog from rushing off and injuring themselves.

* ❧ **recovery.** Slowing your dog's front end with a harness and lead will give their hind legs a better chance to step.

The sling lifts your dog's hindquarters so that they don't collapse or give way. The lead and harness act backwards and towards you to slow your dog and prevent them from dashing off.

Holding a lead and sling at the same time can take getting used to, especially if your dog is wriggly and excitable. Don't worry – it does get easier with practice!

Take your time to get the straps and lead organised in your hands before moving off. Hold the sling in the hand that is nearest to the dog. Hold the lead in your other hand.

The lead acts as brakes. Point it backwards until you feel organised and ready to move off.

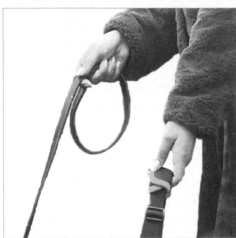

Figure 25: Hold the lead in one hand, and the sling in the other hand.'

Positioning yourself

Position yourself just behind your dog's hindquarters or tail so that you can use the sling in an upward direction.

Watch what your dog is doing. Stop with them when they decide to stop, for example if they choose to sniff the ground.

Walk on your dog's weaker side if they have one. For example, if they tend to knuckle, drag or scuff their right hind paw, walk on their right side. If your dog's hind legs are equally strong, then spend half the time walking on each side.

Slowing your dog during sling walking

Many recovering dogs try to rush ahead, pulling strongly with their front limbs. This might feel like an easy option to your dog. However, it's far better to move slowly:

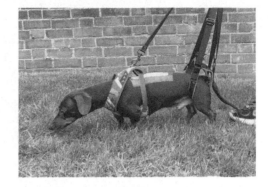

Figure 26: Allow your dog to stop and sniff the ground.

✓ When you slow your dog's front end, their hind legs have a better chance to step.

✓ Slow your dog so that they don't overload and strain their front legs.

Use the lead backwards and towards you to slow your dog.

If your dog sees a cat and tries to make a dash for it, you may need to use the lead quite strongly as brakes. At other times, use the lead with a 'give-take' action: slow your dog for a moment when they lurch forward, then release the pressure a little so that they can travel forward.

Slow your dog's front end. This gives their hind legs a chance to step.

Where to sling-walk your dog

Short grass and artificial turf both give good footing and are unlikely to damage your dog's paws. Bark chips and sand are also good surfaces.

Avoid concrete until your dog can step reliably with their feet the correct way up. Steer clear of shingle or pebbles throughout recovery: stones get between the paw pads, making this a very uncomfortable walking surface.

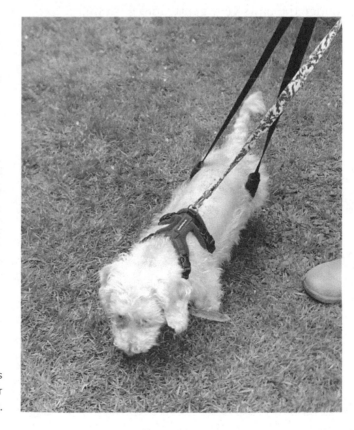

Figure 27: Short grass is an ideal surface for sling walking.

How high to lift the sling

Lift the sling just high enough for your dog's stage of recovery (see figures 28 and 29). Your dog's back should be close to horizontal.

If your dog's rear end is completely floppy, use the sling to support its full weight. This prevents paws getting damaged by trailing along the ground. Their hind paws may brush gently over grass, but when crossing stony ground or concrete, lift a little higher from the sling to avoid damaging their hind paws.

🚫 **AVOID THIS:** Don't let your dog's paws drag over hard ground.

If your dog is trying to step, provide just enough lift from the sling so they don't fall. Allow them to take proper steps.

Correcting your dog's paw position

Now and again, stop and turn your dog's paw(s) the right way up if needed. To do this, put the lead and sling into one hand for a moment, bend over and use your free hand to place each paw the right way up. If unable to bend over, try using a foot to nudge the paws very gently into position.

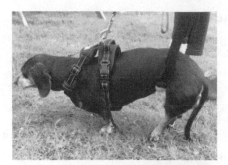

Figure 28 (left): Sling-walking a dog with weak, floppy hind legs.

Figure 29 (below left): Sling-walking a dog that is trying to step with their hind paws.

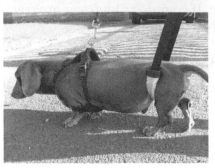

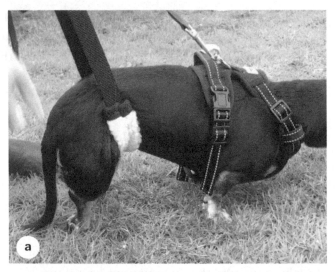

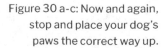
Figure 30 a-c: Now and again, stop and place your dog's paws the correct way up.

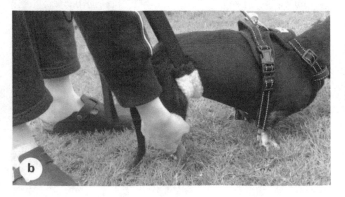

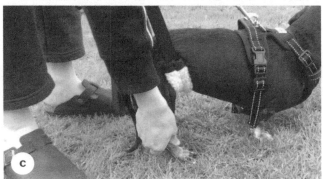

CHAPTER 31
Carrying your dog

You will probably have to lift and carry your dog much more than usual during recovery. Good lifting technique will help protect their back and yours.

Step 1: Preparing to lift your dog

a. A chest harness makes lifting safer. Pop one onto your dog just before lifting, or consider leaving a well-fitting harness on them for a large part of the day (Chapter 26).

b. Get right down to your dog's level if you can. Lower yourself by bending mainly from your knees instead of stooping. This will protect your back, and will avoid alarming your dog by leaning right over them.

c. Talk to your dog and let them know that you are about to lift them. A gentle stroke on the side of the shoulder can help. Steady them from the top of the harness if they are excited or wriggly.

> **TOP TIP:** *Some dogs with back or neck issues might pee without realising it when they are lifted. Protect your clothes by tucking an old towel under your dog's rear end just before lifting.*

Step 2: Lifting and carrying

How to carry your dog depends on their size and shape and on what feels most comfortable to both of you.

Smaller dogs

a. Support their chest with one hand, and use your other hand or arm to support their rear end.

b. As you lift, bring your dog towards your chest to help keep them steady. Tuck at least one finger into your dog's chest harness for added security in case they wriggle.

BOX 8: LIFTING AND CARRYING **SUMMARY**

✓ Plan the route in advance.

✓ Use both hands.

✓ Support your dog's front and rear ends.

✓ For safety:
- hold the dog close to your body.
- loop a finger into their chest harness.

✓ Take care of your own back (see box 9).

BOX 9: CARRYING A DACHSHUND

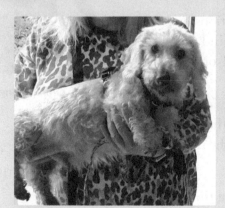

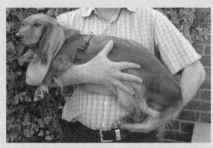

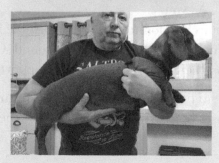

The best way to carry a dachshund depends on their size and on what feels comfortable to both of you.

Support them under both the chest and rump. Hold your dog close against your chest to support the length of their back. Use one or both forearms for extra support.

Larger dogs

a. Support your larger dog with two arms. Wrap one arm around the front of the chest, and the other behind their rump.

b. Tuck your dog in close to your body as you lift.

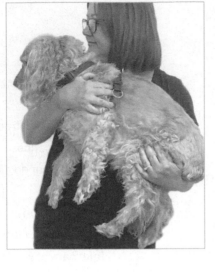
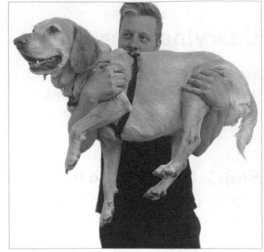

Figure 32: Lifting a larger dog.

Lifting with two people

Each person has their own limit for lifting. If your dog is heavier than 15-20 kg, you will probably need help to lift them.

Decide who should carry which end of the dog, bearing in mind that the front end is usually slightly heavier than the rear. Plan your route before you start. Check that any doors are open and that footing is safe. Squat down at floor level on one side of the dog. Organise yourselves before you start to lift:

🐾 The person at the head end positions one arm under the dog's ribcage behind the front legs, and the other arm in front of the dog's chest.

🐾 The person at the rear end places one arm under the dog's belly in front of the hind legs, and the other arm behind the dog's rump.

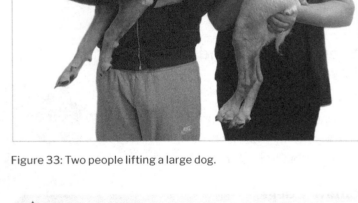

Figure 33: Two people lifting a large dog.

⚠ **WATCH OUT:** Don't let either end of your dog dangle unsupported.

Agree to lift together after a count of three, for example "one, two, three, LIFT". As you each lift, bring the dog in close to your chest for added support. Agree in advance where you are taking the dog and how they will be positioned after lowering to the ground. On reaching your destination, lower the dog gently, either resting on their front or side or in a supported standing position.

Very large dogs require three people to lift. The chest and rump are supported by two people as described above. The third person uses both arms to support under the dog's belly.

Step 3: Lowering your dog

a. Support your dog's front and rear ends as you lower them to the ground.

b. Prop your dog in a stable, natural-looking position before you let go of them. You could lay them on their front or on one side if very weak. Stronger dogs may be helped into a sitting or standing position before you let go. Give as much support as needed before you take your hands away.

 ADVANCED TIP: If possible, help your dog touch down gently with their hind paws before their front paws. Even if your dog is paralysed, this will help their recovery by reminding them of their normal coordination pattern. As you do this, continue to support the chest and rump until your dog is securely carrying their own weight.

BOX 10: LOOKING AFTER YOUR OWN BACK WHILE LIFTING

Your dog needs you to stay safe! Take care of your own back.

✓ Plan ahead

- If your dog is too heavy for you to manage easily, get help.

- Before you start, prop doors open, and check for any twists, turns and steps within the route.

- Check your footwear. High heels or flip-flops make lifting difficult.

- Place low stools or floor cushions at the start and end of the route if these will help you to get down to floor level.

✓ Lift with good technique

- Keep your feet around shoulder width apart.

- Get down by bending mainly from the legs. Don't stoop.

- Use your arms to support your dog close to your body.

- Start to lift your dog, then straighten your legs to get upright.

- Don't turn and lift at the same time. If you need to turn, do so once you are already upright.

 WARNING: Consult a doctor if you're worried.

CHAPTER 32

'Together time' – sitting safely with your dog

Many dogs expect regular close contact with their owntetrs. During 'together time', your dog can sit, lie or try to stand next to you, while you take care to keep them safe. They must not wander off or fall.

Sitting on the floor

If you can get down to floor level, sit on the floor with your dog next to you on carpet or non-slip matting.

> **Keep a hold of their chest harness even when you are relaxing together.**

Dogs sometimes rush off unpredictably in response to the doorbell or for no apparent reason.

Sitting on the sofa

Some owners find it difficult to get down to floor level and prefer to sit with their dog on their lap or on the sofa. These dogs are liable to lurch off unexpectedly and injure themselves. They could also slip into an awkward position between sofa cushions. Use blankets or towels if needed to block off gaps between sofa cushions.

 WARNING: Only consider putting your dog on the sofa if you are prepared to keep hold of their chest harness.

Keeping your dog calm

Pay attention to what your dog is doing. They might try to get up and move around if people enter the room, or if they hear noises from outside. Calm them as needed, and steady them from their harness. A palm at the front of their chest can help to stop them inching forward (see Figure 35b).

→ **See Chapter 39 'Confidence building techniques' for more details.**

If your dog is too restless, put them back in their crate or pen to allow them to settle down.

> ### SAFETY ADVICE
>
> **Sitting with your dog**
>
> ✓ Have them wear a chest harness (see Chapter 26, 'Your dog's harness').
>
> ✓ Keep your fingers tucked into their harness whenever they are sitting with you outside the recovery crate or pen.
>
> ✓ Check that your dog's footing is non-slip and gives good safe support.
>
> ✓ If you need to leave the room for a moment, return the dog to their crate until you return.
>
> ✗ If your dog is on a sofa or other raised surface, don't take your hands off them, even for a moment.

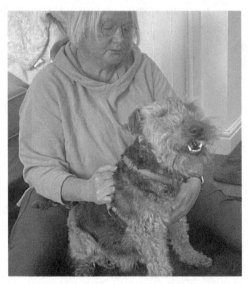

Figure 34 (top): Sitting on the floor with a dog.

Figure 35a (middle) and b (bottom): Always keep hold of your dog's harness if they are on a sofa.

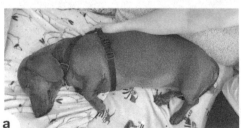

a

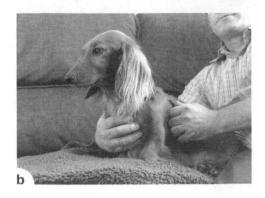

b

CHAPTER 33

Caring for your dog's surgical wound

After spinal surgery, the wound or surgical site must be kept clean so that it can heal. Some wounds are held together by absorbable sutures (stitches) hidden under the surface. Others have visible sutures or staples which must be removed at your dog's usual vet practice at around 10-14 days after the operation.

Keeping an eye on the wound

Once the dressing has been removed or has fallen off, check the surgical site at least once daily. It should look clean and its edges should be holding together. Ask your vet for advice if you notice one or more of the following around the wound:

- swelling
- unpleasant smell
- red skin
- smelly or persistent discharge
- wound edges gaping

Protecting the wound

Your dog must not lick at the wound until it has healed (usually 10-14 days). It may only take a few seconds for them to remove stitches or staples or to introduce infection.

KEY POINTS

✓ Check the wound at least daily until healed (10-14 days). Report any concerns to your vet.

✓ Use an Elizabethan collar or surgical vest if needed to prevent your dog from licking or damaging the area.

✗ Don't bathe your dog or allow the surgical incision to get wet until it has healed.

✗ Don't apply any creams or disinfectants to the wound unless your vet has asked you to do so.

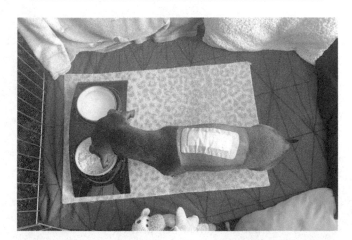

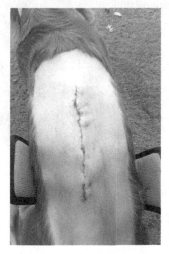
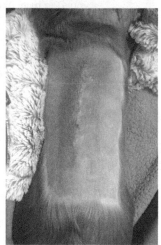

Figure 36 (top): There may be a light dressing over the wound when your dog first comes home.

Figure 37: A healthy wound at (a) 7 days (above left) and (b) 3 weeks (above right) after surgery. In some dogs, fur starts to grow back sooner than this.

A plastic Elizabethan collar (cone) gives the most reliable protection, so use this 24 hours a day if your dog is determined to get at the area. However, after spinal surgery, many dogs find an inflatable collar, surgical vest, or fabric cone more comfortable than a plastic cone. Ask the vet or nurse for advice when your dog comes home.

 TIP: *If your dog is wearing a cone, check that they can still access food and water easily. You may need to use a smaller bowl or to raise the bowl slightly.*

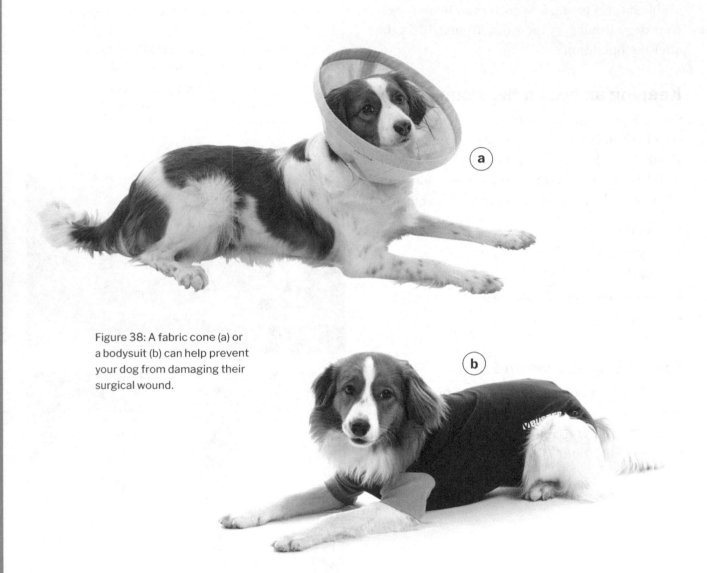

Figure 38: A fabric cone (a) or a bodysuit (b) can help prevent your dog from damaging their surgical wound.

SECTION 6
Your dog's wellbeing

This section explains how to keep your dog happy and content during recovery.

CHAPTER 34
Keeping your dog happy at home during recovery

Recovering dogs cannot be expected to understand why their life has suddenly changed. They can't go for their usual walks, jump on the sofa or play with balls. It's no wonder that some find the recovery period a challenge. Luckily, there is plenty that you can do to make life more pleasant for your furry friend during recovery.

Make their recovery area comfortable

The crate, pen or recovery room is your dog's own little world for much of the day and night, so it is essential to make it comfortable.

Enough space

Check that your dog's crate or pen is big enough. They need enough space to stretch out fully for comfort.

→ **See chapter 18, 'Crate or pen size'**

Bedding

Offer plenty of bedding and block off any draughts if needed. This will encourage rest.

→ **See chapter 22, 'Your dog's bedding'**

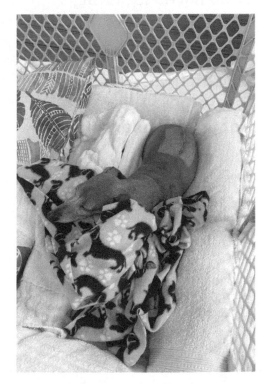

Figure 1: Check that your dog's crate or pen is comfortable.

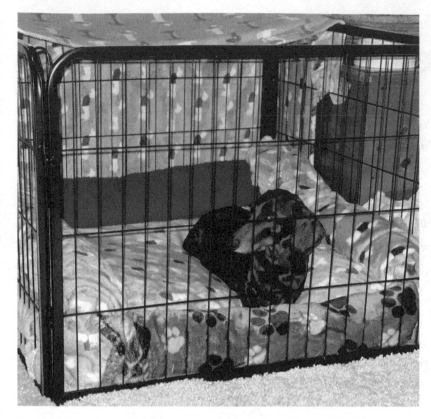

Figure 2: Covering part of the crate or pen can help a dog to settle down.

Check the position of the crate or pen

Some dogs love to be in the busiest area of the house so that they can see, hear and smell what is going on at all times. Others get upset by the comings and goings of people and other dogs nearby. If household bustle and noise seem to be making your dog anxious, consider having them recover in a quieter part of the home.

→ **See Chapter 19, 'Where to put the crate or pen'**

TIP: *If you dog wants to be part of the family, but also likes a bit of privacy, try covering part of their crate or pen with a sheet or blanket.*

Adaptil products

Dog Appeasing Pheromone (DAP) is produced by mother dogs to help their pups feel more content and calm. Adaptil is a synthetic form of this chemical available as a diffuser, spray or collar. Try plugging the diffuser in very close to your dog's crate, or try using the spray on bedding in the crate.

Leave the radio playing

Try leaving the radio or recorded music playing at certain times of the day to help your dog settle down. Studies have found that recordings of gentle classical music or soft reggae may have a calming effect on some dogs. Remember that your confined dog cannot escape from noise, so set the music no louder than a gentle speaking volume.

Set up a regular routine

Make a regular daily routine for your recovering dog. They will feel calmer if they know what to expect. The best routine depends mainly on your dog's stage of recovery and on whether they can walk.

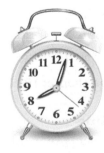

For general advice see:

❖ Chapter 10 if your dog can walk

❖ Chapters 12-14 if your dog cannot walk

→ **Examples of daily routines can be found in Appendix 1.**

CHAPTER 35
Toys

Help your recovering dog feel better by offering suitable toys in their crate or pen. Always follow the safety guidelines (see box 1).

Food-dispensing toys

Dogs love to lick and chew at things. The challenge of getting food out of food dispensing toys can help to keep them absorbed. You can even feed their entire food ration from food-dispensers instead of from a bowl.

 TIP: *Fill food-dispensers using your dog's usual food ration and daily treat allowance.* Dogs get overweight if they eat too much peanut butter or other high calorie foods.

→ **See Chapter 80, 'How much to feed'.**

Only choose food-dispensers that your dog will use calmly. Two of the safest types during early recovery are the lick mats and snuffle mats.

Lick mat

This textured rubber mat can be smeared with wet dog food, liver paste or mashed cooked carrot or apple. Place it on the crate floor or fix vertically at your dog's head height. Lick mats are also useful for keeping dogs focused at exercise time (Chapters 58-59).

After use, some types can go in the dishwasher, while others must be scrubbed clean with a brush and soapy water.

 TIP: *Pureed vegetables are a good low-calorie option for filling the lick mat.* Boil or microwave them, then batch-freeze in an ice cube tray for future use.

Snuffle mat

Place this on the floor of your dog's crate or pen, and tuck in pieces of kibble, dry treats or slivers of raw carrot for them to find. You must keep the mat clean, so look for a machine washable one.

> **SAFETY ADVICE**
>
> ### Box 1: Toys –
> ### Safety guidelines
>
> **Don't let your dog eat the toy or choke on parts of it**
>
> ✓ Supervise them, especially when offering anything new.
>
> ✓ Remove damaged toys.
>
> ✓ Choose toys designed for your dog's size.
>
> **Only offer toys that your dog will settle down with calmly**
>
> ✗ Avoid balls and other rolling toys.
>
> ✗ Don't give your dog anything that you expect them to shake violently.
>
> ✗ Avoid items that they might throw and chase.

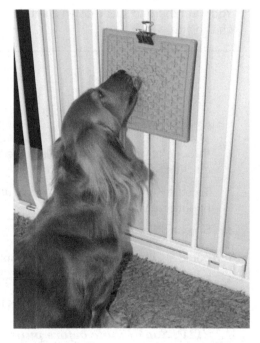

Figure 3 (above): A lick mat in use – dogs enjoy working for food!

Figure 4 (below): The snuffle mat is suitable for most dogs during early recovery.

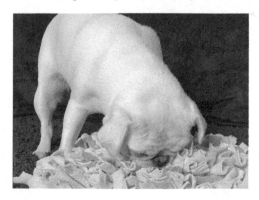

Kong

A Kong is a hollow rubber toy that can be filled with food to challenge your dog.

Using Kongs safely **SAFETY ADVICE**

⚠ **TAKE CARE!** Kongs cause some dogs to get too excited. Check with your vet before starting to use them. Kongs are usually best avoided until at least 3 weeks into IVDD recovery.

✓ Choose a Kong that is designed for your dog's size and chewing ability. If it's too small or flimsy it could become a choking hazard.

✓ Keep an eye on your dog.

✓ Place the filled Kong gently into your dog's crate or pen instead of throwing or rolling it at them.

You want them to settle down quietly with the Kong instead of chasing it.

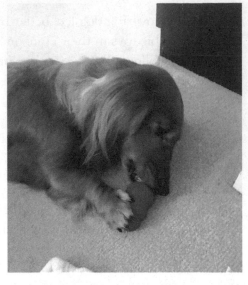

Figure 5: Dogs enjoy getting food out of a Kong.

BOX 3: FILLING A KONG

1. Put one of your dog's treats into the Kong. This could be a dog biscuit, piece of cooked chicken or long sliver of carrot.

2. Top the Kong up with your dog's usual food. If using kibble, soak it first for about 10 minutes in water.

3. Smear wet dog food or mashed cooked carrot or apple over the top of the Kong to seal it.

You could also turn this into a Kong ice lolly:

4. Put the filled Kong in a bag in the freezer for 4 hours.

5. Wipe the Kong with a damp cloth before handing to your dog.

 TIP: *Soak kibble before putting it into the Kong. Dry kibble might scatter everywhere and cause your dog to rush about.*

After each use, clean the Kong either in the dishwasher or by hand.

Interactive games

Some food dispensing toys are designed to challenge the dog's intelligence. To reach the food, they must rotate, slide, or lift parts of the toy in a certain order.

Use these puzzles as interactive games instead of leaving your dog alone with them. Sit on the floor with your dog and help them get started – you may need to show them what to do at each stage so they don't get frustrated.

Only offer these games on non-slip flooring. Use your hands, if needed, to help prop your dog's hindquarters as they play. They may need to use their front paws in solving the puzzle.

Soft toys

Only offer soft toys if you expect your dog to interact with them calmly. It's fine for them to pick toys up and to move them about gently.

⚠️ **WATCH OUT!** Avoid soft toys if your dog is likely to shake them violently. This applies to many dachshunds and terriers.

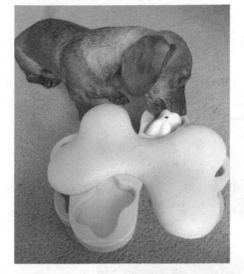

Figure 6 (left): Tornado, an interactive toy from Nina Ottossen. The dog must rotate some shapes and lift others to reach the food.

Figure 7 (below): Twister, an interactive toy from Nina Ottossen.

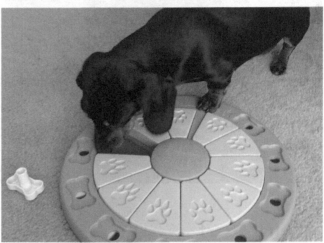

If your dog has several toys, offer them on rotation. Some owners find that using three or more different toys on daily rotation helps to keep their dog's interest.

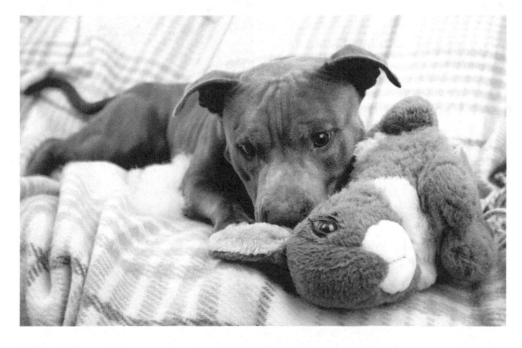

Figure 8: Dogs are most comforted by items that smell familiar. Use your dog's old toys instead of buying new ones.

CHAPTER 36

Dog pushchairs

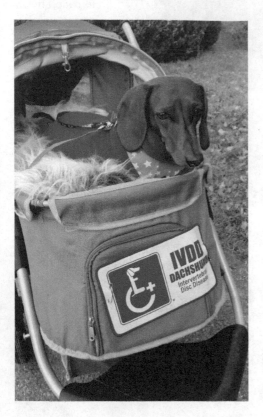

A pushchair (stroller) will be useful if your dog's recovery is expected to take more than a few weeks. This is a safe way for them to reach old familiar places and to sniff somewhere new. Lift your dog out for their prescribed amount of timed lead exercise, then put them back in the chair to rest.

⚠ **TAKE CARE:** For safety, clip your dog's harness to the pushchair during use, and always keep a close eye on them.

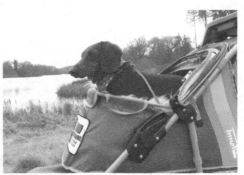

Figure 9 (far left): Many recovering dogs enjoy pushchair rides.

Figure 10 (left): If your dog feels the cold, have them wear a jacket or cover them with a blanket in the colder months.

When to start

You can normally start short pushchair rides from two weeks after surgery or injury. If you don't have a garden and need to wheel your dog to a safe patch of grass, you may be able to start sooner. Check first with your vet.

 TIP: *If your dog is weak, stabilise them by placing a rolled blanket on either side.*

Introducing your dog to the pushchair

1. Start indoors. Place your dog in the pushchair, clip them in using their harness, and hand them treats if needed to get their confidence up.
2. Outdoors, make the first pushchair journey no longer than ten minutes.
3. Build up the length of the pushchair rides gradually over several weeks.

Make your dog's first ride in the pushchair no longer than ten minutes.

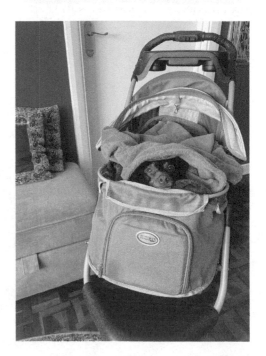

Figure 11: Have your dog try the pushchair indoors first

CHAPTER 37
Understanding what your dog is thinking

Dogs mainly communicate using body language

As you interact with your dog during recovery, watch their body language carefully. You can then adjust what you are doing to help them feel better.

A healthy, happy, relaxed dog moves freely and fluidly. When they're very active, their mouth may be slightly open, tongue perhaps lolling to one side (see figure 12). When resting, their face looks relaxed (see figure 13). An anxious dog may instead turn their head or body away, tuck their tail between their hind legs, and get up and leave or try to hide.

During recovery from IVDD, pain and difficulty moving can leave dogs feeling more vulnerable than usual. They may also find it difficult to communicate normally. Unlike a healthy dog, they cannot move freely or get up and leave, and they may be unable to turn their body normally or use their tail for communication.

It's essential to watch your dog for more subtle body language.

Calming signals (signs of unease)

In both sickness and health, dogs use calming signals to let other dogs or people know when they feel stressed or uneasy (see box 4). Watch carefully for these signs. For example, an overwhelmed or anxious dog may try to tell you this by licking their lips (fig 14) or by yawning (figure 15). Of course, dogs also yawn when they're tired or lick their lips after eating. But if these signals happen during an interaction with someone it usually means the dog is feeling uneasy.

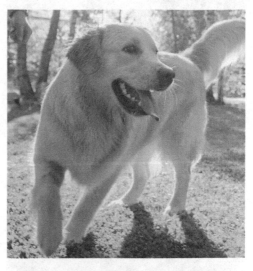

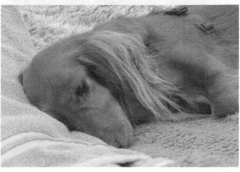

Figure 12 (top): A happy, relaxed healthy dog.

Figure 13 (above): A dog enjoying gentle home massage. The muscles around her eyes are soft and relaxed.

Dogs use calming signals, such as yawning or lip-licking, to tell us that they are feeling anxious.

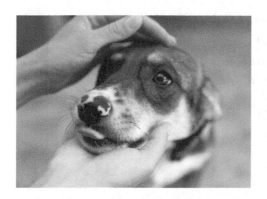

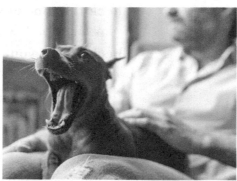

Figure 14 (far left): Lip-licking.

Figure 15 (left): Yawning can be a sign of anxiety in dogs.

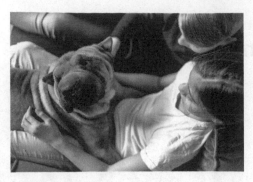

Figure 16: This dog is turning his head away from the children as he feels a little too crowded.

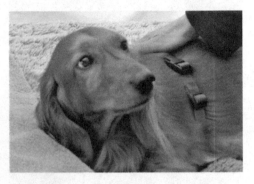

Figure 17: This dog feels slightly uneasy. The muscles around her eyes and mouth are tense.

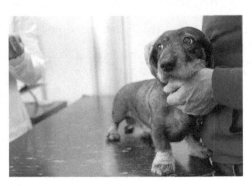

Figure 18: A tense, anxious dog.

BOX 4: CALMING SIGNALS

Dogs tend to show that they feel overwhelmed, uneasy or anxious by doing one or more of the following:

- Lip-licking – a very quick flicking movement of their tongue (figure 14)
- Yawning (figure 15)
- Blinking their eyes rapidly
- Turning their head or body away from someone (figure 16)
- Wagging their tail while also looking frightened
- Lifting a front paw
- Looking tense in their face while showing the whites of their eyes (figures 17 and 18)
- Freezing – going unexpectedly still

Some anxious dogs also try to distract themselves by:

- sniffing the ground
- licking the floor or licking one of their legs
- scratching themselves

What to do if your dog shows calming signals or looks anxious

If your dog yawns or uses another calming signal, pause for a moment and check what you are doing.

- ❧ **Don't crowd your dog.** During recovery, dogs can get anxious if we bend right over them, hug them tight, gaze into their eyes or get too close to their face (for example by kissing them on the nose). Reposition yourself if needed so that your dog feels less crowded.

- ❧ **Slow your movements down.** Dogs can feel overwhelmed if people are in too much of a hurry, for example when putting their harness on, cleaning or massaging them. Pause now and again to give your dog more time to process what is happening.

- ❧ **Check the tone of your voice.** Your dog may get worried if someone sounds angry.

- ❧ **Check where your hands are on your dog.** Touching over a tight muscle or other sore spot might leave them feeling uneasy.

What does whining mean?

Some dogs whine while greeting people or other dogs. This can either mean that they are excited or anxious.

If your dog is whining when left in their crate or pen, this suggests one or more of the following:

1. **Your dog needs something.** They may be trying to tell you that something is wrong. Perhaps they have knocked the water bowl over. Or maybe the room is too cold, the next meal is due, or they need to be taken outside to pee. Your dog might mix some barking in with this type of whining.

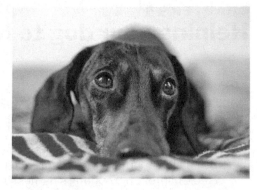

Figure 19: Dogs can whine for many different reasons.

2. **Pain.** A dog that is unsettled or anxious due to pain may whine frequently. Expect to see other signs of discomfort if the whining is mainly due to pain (see chapter 42, 'Is my dog in pain?'). The whining may get worse, or turn into moaning or yelping, whenever the dog tries to change position.

3. **Attention-seeking.** Constant or frequent whining while coming to the front of the crate and looking for their owner usually suggests that the dog is trying to get attention. This whining may get more intense as you enter the room. Whining may be interspersed with barking or little yips. These dogs usually look alert, with head up and big, appealing eyes.

Recognising when a dog may be about to bite

It's very unusual for a dog to bite with no warning. Instead, most dogs try to tell us that they are feeling anxious or overwhelmed. They usually start by showing subtle calming signals (signs of unease) such as yawning or lip-licking. On becoming increasingly anxious, they may try to get away from the situation by struggling or trying to move away.

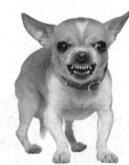

Figure 20: Growling is a dog's way of telling us to back off. Always respect this.

Growling. A dog that is growling feels very distressed and may try to bite if people approach. While growling, dogs tend to look tense and stiff, perhaps staring directly at someone or showing the whites of their eyes. They may also bare their teeth or snap at the air.

TIP: *Never tell a dog off for growling.* This only makes them feel worse. In fact, growling is a useful signal that shows us how the dog is feeling. A dog that is scolded for growling may go on in future to bite without warning.

What does a waggy tail mean?

During a bout of IVDD, some dogs cannot move their tail much or at all. So, from a recovery point of view, it's generally good news if your dog can wag their tail.

Having said that, for those that can use their tail, don't read too much into any tail-wagging.

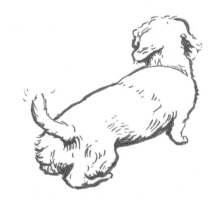

Dogs wag their tails when they are excited, for example on greeting a favourite person. However, a wagging tail doesn't always indicate happiness. It can also mean that they are playful, anxious or frightened. Watch the rest of their body to get a clearer idea of how they are feeling.

CHAPTER 38
Helping your dog to feel more confident

BOX 5: GENTLE HANDLING

✓ Slow down: Give your dog enough time to process what is happening.

✓ Use a chest harness for support and restraint (see Chapter 26 'Your dog's harness')

✓ Support your dog with two hands if you need to move them (see Chapter 31 'Carrying your dog')

✓ Watch and respond to your dog's body language (see Chapter 37 'Understanding what your dog is thinking')

 WHAT TO DO If your dog is anxious about what you are doing with them:

• pause and adjust your position

• breathe deeply, then start again more slowly

• or stop for a while.

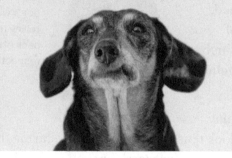

Why we need gentle handling during recovery

This can feel like a difficult time for your dog. They might be uncomfortable, uncoordinated and easily knocked off-balance. To make matters worse, their routine has just been turned upside-down. Handle them gently and positively to leave them feeling more relaxed, confident and comfortable.

Whether helping your dog in or out of the crate, lifting them, doing prescribed massage or anything else, remember to have 'kind hands'. Do your best to avoid gripping your dog rigidly, or digging your fingertips into them, both of which can hurt and put your dog on edge.

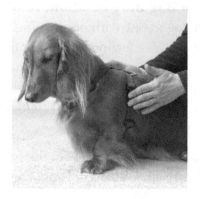

Figure 22: Always remember to have 'kind hands'.

Stay positive

Our canine friends are quick to pick up on our emotions. Even if you are having a bad day, do your best to stay positive whenever talking to or handling them. This can make a big difference to how your dog feels, especially if you are their favourite person.

IVDD recovery can certainly feel like a challenge. For tips on caring for yourself through recovery, see Section 16, 'Your wellbeing'.

Check the tone of your voice

Speak kindly to your dog rather than snapping or shouting at them. The tone of your voice is more important than what you say.

✓ To encourage your dog to wake up and come with you, try an upbeat, higher-pitched voice.

✓ Speak in a slower, more soothing tone to encourage them to calm down.

Use rewards instead of punishments

The recovery period may be a learning process for your dog. For example they might need to learn not to dash past you out of their crate.

Whenever your dog does something good, reward them immediately by saying "good boy/girl" in a kind voice. Offer a small food reward at the same time if needed. This helps your dog learn to cooperate with you.

If your dog does something unacceptable, you can say "no" simply and firmly. Be sure to reward them as soon as they do the right thing.

Avoid shouting at your dog or getting cross. Remember they're confined and so cannot go off and hide. If you feel full of bottled-up frustration, put them safely into the crate and then leave the room until you have calmed down.

How to position yourself when handling your dog

Try to face the same way as your dog when doing anything that might make them anxious such as sponge bathing or checking their surgical wound. This should help to put them at ease.

Humans usually greet one another face to face and make direct eye contact, but dogs naturally find this approach rather awkward. Try approaching your dog from the side rather than from directly in front.

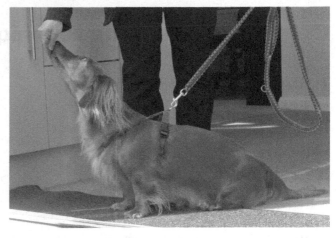

Figure 23: Reward your dog for good behaviour.

BOX 6: POSITIONING YOURSELF

✓ Face the same way as your dog whenever doing something that might make them anxious, for example when checking their surgical wound.

✓ Don't crowd your recovering dog. They might find it overwhelming:

✗ don't stare directly into their eyes.

✗ avoid leaning right across them.

✗ avoid loose scarves or jewellery that could dangle over them during handling.

✗ do your best not to smother their face with kisses!

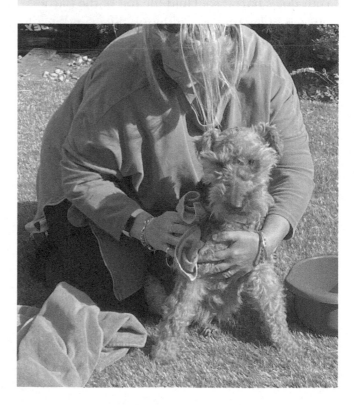

Figure 24: Facing the same way as your dog can help put them at ease.

CHAPTER 39
Confidence-building techniques

1. Steady from the top of the harness

Use this technique for safety and to improve your dog's confidence. Steady them from the top of their harness to keep their bodyweight safely over all four paws.

When?

✓ To stop your dog rushing off

- When sitting with your dog outside the pen
- During any care-giving procedure at home or in the clinic

✓ To steady your dog and get their attention:

- As you greet them
- Before lifting and carrying
- Just before you clip their lead onto the harness

✓ Your dog can be sitting, standing or lying.

How?

Put a chest harness on your dog (see Chapter 26, 'Your dog's harness'). Hold the top of the harness between index finger and thumb. Slow and steady them as needed from the harness top. Respond to what your dog does. As they start to move forward, apply gentle backward pressure from the harness to steady their bodyweight over all four paws. This stops them from lurching forward and gives their paws better control.

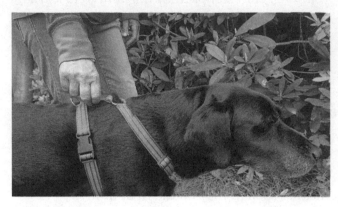

Figure 25: Steadying a dog from the top of their harness.

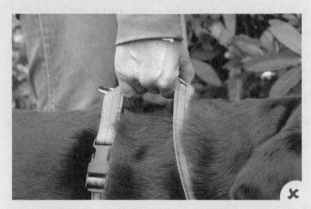

BOX 7: BIRD BEAK HOLD

✗ **AVOID** holding the harness like a suitcase handle. This could swing your dog off-balance.

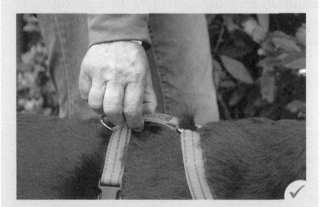

✓ **BIRD BEAK HOLD.** Instead, think of your index finger and thumb coming together on the harness like a bird's beak. This slows and steadies the dog more precisely. If it's more comfortable for you, or if you need extra control, use all your fingers.

2. Palm at the front of the chest

This simple technique can be used on any dog but is particularly useful for breeds such as dachshunds that have a prominent keel (breastbone) at the front of the chest. It can help to soothe and steady them, even during the worst of their spinal pain.

When?

✓ To prevent your dog from rushing forward

- While sitting with them indoors or in the garden
- During any care-giving procedures such as sponge bathing
- Between exercises

✓ To calm an excitable or painful dog

- At home
- At the clinic, in the waiting room or on the vet's table

✓ Your dog can be sitting, standing or lying on their front

How?

Position yourself either next to or behind your dog, facing the same way as them. Spread your palm and place it gently at the front of their chest.

If your dog tries to rush forward, use your hand as a brake.

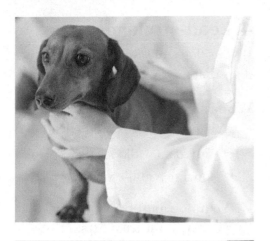

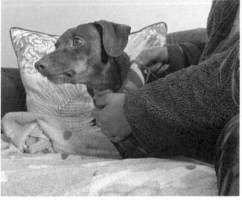

Figure 27 (top): A palm at the front of your dog's chest can be soothing.

Figure 28 (above): Try using 'Palm at the front of the chest' while steadying your dog from the top of the harness. This gives extra support.

3. Hands around your dog's shoulders

This is another technique to calm a dog and to help prevent them from rushing forward.

When?

✓ As for 'Palm at the front of the chest' (see no. 2 above)
✓ Very useful in broad-chested breeds such as French bulldogs.

How?

Position yourself either next to or behind your dog, and facing the same way as them. Wrap both hands gently around their shoulders (figure 29). Think of your hands as being 'soft' and avoid grabbing at your dog or digging fingertips into their skin.

Steady your dog with your hands if they start to barge forward or sideways.

⚠ **WATCH OUT: This technique does not leave a hand free to hold your dog's harness.** Link your fingers into their harness for added security if needed.

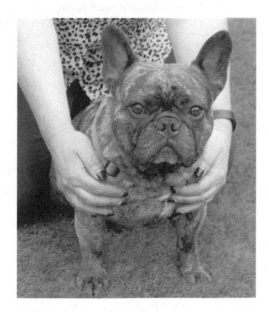

Figure 29: Contain your dog with soft hands around their shoulders.

4. Lead-stroking

If your dog can stand and walk a little, you can use lead stroking as a calming technique. It's useful for dogs that are anxious, excited or uncomfortable.

When?

✓ When your dog is on the lead. They can be either standing or sitting.

- Out on a walk, for example while you pause to talk to someone
- During a clinic visit, for a few seconds at a time when your dog is on the floor.

✓ Your dog must be on harness and lead.

✗ Don't try this when sling-walking. You need two hands on the lead for this technique.

How?

Before you start: Hold the lead with two hands as shown in box 8 and in Chapter 29, 'Using the lead'. Position yourself next to your dog's hindquarters and face the same way as your dog. The lead should point backwards from its clip.

Method: Stroke slowly along the lead towards your body with alternate hands. This action is similar to hauling in a rope, but much more gentle. Stroke as lightly as is needed, without tipping your dog off-balance.

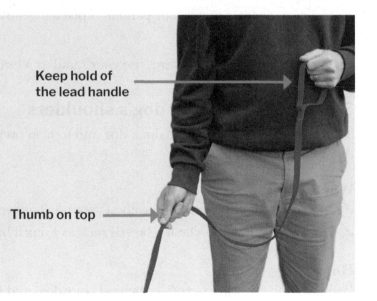

BOX 8: HOLDING THE LEAD FOR LEAD-STROKING

One hand holds the lead handle. The other hand holds the lead itself, thumb on top of the lead and pointing down the lead towards the dog.

 TIP: As you stroke along the lead, keep the lead handle tucked into one hand so it doesn't dangle and distract your dog.

Keep hold of the lead handle

Thumb on top

Learning this technique

Get confident with lead-stroking by trying it without your dog to start with. Either have a friend hold the clip end of the lead, or attach it to a chair leg. Try stroking along the lead as shown in the pictures.

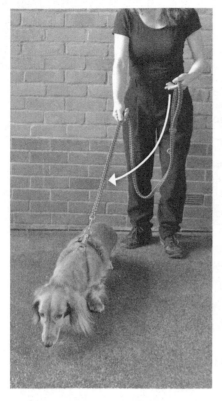

Figure 30a: Left hand moves in the direction of the white arrow, while still holding the lead handle.

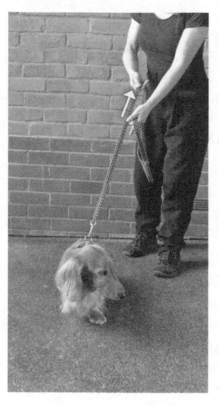

Figure 30b: Left hand slides up the lead in the direction of the yellow arrow.

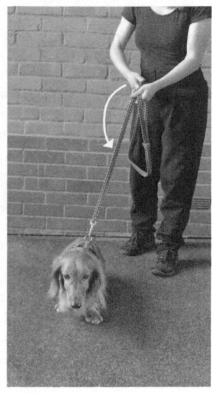

Figure 30c: Right hand comes off the lead and travels in the direction of the white arrow.

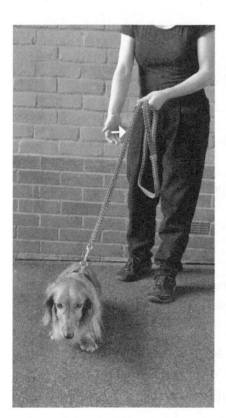

Figure 30d: Take hold of the lead again with your right hand, palm facing upward.

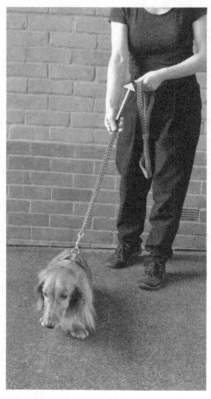

Figure 30e: Right hand slides up the lead in the direction of the yellow arrow.

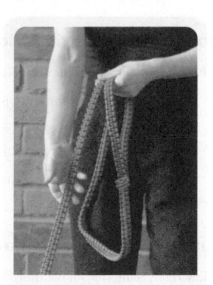

⚠ **CHECK THIS:** Your palm must go **under** the lead for lead-stroking to work as a calming technique.

CHAPTER 40
Anxious dogs: Getting further help

Some dogs are anxious during recovery and need special care. A sore back or neck can leave them feeling unsettled, as can the big change of routine that happens during a bout of IVDD.

In the first instance, the best person to advise you is your vet (see box 9).

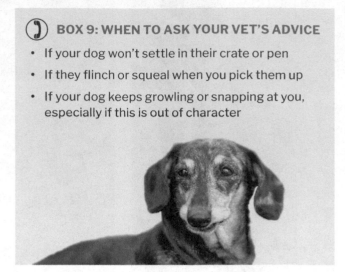

BOX 9: WHEN TO ASK YOUR VET'S ADVICE

- If your dog won't settle in their crate or pen
- If they flinch or squeal when you pick them up
- If your dog keeps growling or snapping at you, especially if this is out of character

Medication to help an anxious dog through recovery

Anxiety and pain often go together. Your vet can assess your dog for pain and adjust their painkillers as needed. They may also decide to prescribe something to help your dog feel less anxious. For example, trazadone tablets are sometimes prescribed together with certain painkillers to help dogs feel better during their crate rest period.

If your dog will not settle in their crate, it is generally not a good idea to try and solve the problem by giving strong sedatives. A dog that is heavily sedated may still feel anxious or painful, but now they are left feeling helpless too.

Home care for anxious dogs

While any medication starts to take effect, give your dog special care at home to leave them feeling better:

1. Check that their pen or crate is comfortable (Section 4)

2. Fit your dog with a harness (Chapter 26) so that you don't need to pull on their neck collar or to grab their body when restraining them.

3. Try the confidence-building techniques described in Chapter 39 when you need to get hands-on with your dog.

Further help from a behaviourist

A few recovering dogs have more severe or complex behavioural problems. Discuss this with your vet and consider asking them to refer you to a qualified canine behaviourist. This is someone with at least degree level training in animal behaviour.

- In the UK, look for those registered with the organisations ABTC, FABC, ASAB, APBC, or for a vet with specialist or advanced practitioner status in animal behaviour.
- In the US, a behaviourist should have one of the following qualifications: CAAB, ACAAB or DipACVB.

The behaviourist can assess the situation, find out why your dog is feeling distressed, and give you bespoke advice including practical ways to resolve the problem.

CHAPTER 41
Troubleshooting

My dog won't stop crying

If only animals could talk! Dogs may cry during crate rest for several reasons. They could be feeling painful, or they may be unsettled because they are too cold or they need to go to pee or poo. Or they may be bored or just keen to get your attention.

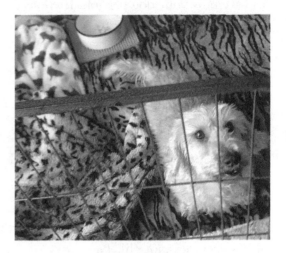

Figure 31: Dogs may try to get our attention for various reasons. This dog needed to get outdoors to the toilet.

First check the following:

1. Try taking them out to the toilet if they have not been recently.

2. Check that your dog can reach their water. If they can't move, prop them up and hold the bowl under their chin now and again for a chance to drink.

3. Does your dog flinch or squeal on being lifted or when they try to move? If so, they might need painkillers prescribed, or doses adjusted. Ask your vet's advice. For other possible signs of pain, see Chapter 42, 'Is my dog in pain?'.

4. Is the crate comfortable? Check that it is large enough for your dog to stretch out, and block off any draughts. Try covering half of the crate with a sheet to help them settle down.

5. Does your dog have enough to do? Try dividing their daily ration between food dispensing toys. The snuffle mat and lick mat are safest during early recovery (Chapter 35).

> **ASK YOUR VET'S ADVICE** if your dog does not settle down within a day or two of following the advice on this page. They might need to adjust your dog's painkiller regime or prescribe something to reduce anxiety.

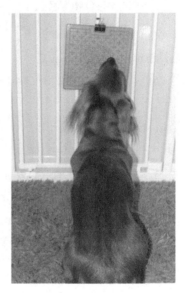

Figure 32: A lick mat can be used from early recovery to give your dog something to do.

Further practical tips to help your dog settle down:

✓ Set up a regular daily routine that includes all their basic daily needs (see Appendix 1, 'Routines').

✓ When checking on your dog:
  • Keep your voice calm, quiet, and unemotional so as not to appear to 'reward' them for crying.
  • Avoid the temptation to shout at your crying dog, as this causes upset and confusion and may make the crying worse.
  • During the night, keep the lights dim and your voice low. Your dog needs to learn not to expect attention at certain times of the day and night.

✗ Don't hand food or toys to your dog while they are crying.
  • Wait for a break in the noise before handing them anything.
  • Give them a little food or a toy whenever you return them to the crate or pen. This will make them feel better about going in there.

Some dogs settle down better if the crate is in a quiet room, while others prefer to be surrounded by their family in a living room or kitchen-diner area. If nothing else is working, consider moving the crate and see how your dog gets on. If your crate-rested dog wants to be surrounded by family, set up an extra crate so that they can be moved around the house with you. For example, consider having one in your living area and another in your bedroom.

Help, my dog is biting me!

Why might dogs bite?

Dogs occasionally bite out of pain or fear. This can happen if an IVDD dog is very painful on being picked up. A recent memory of pain could also cause some dogs to get uneasy and to bite when they are next handled. Those that are not used to close handling may feel overwhelmed by hands-on procedures.

Many dogs with back or neck problems cannot move away or would find it painful to do so. If we ignore signs of anxiety and grab the dog or hold them down for a procedure, they get more distressed and biting becomes more likely.

What to do

🗨 **ASK YOUR VET.** If your dog is growling, snapping or biting, and if this is out of character, they may be in pain. Ask to speak to your vet. They can check that your dog's pain medication is sufficient.

In the meantime...

If exercises, massage or range of movement cause growling or snapping then stop doing them for now, and ask advice from the vet or physiotherapist who prescribed them.

You still need to handle your dog for essential tasks such as getting them out to the toilet and expressing their bladder if needed.

- **Leave a well-fitting harness on them.** You can easily steady or restrain your dog by getting hold of the top of the harness, or by clipping a lead to it.
- **Watch for subtle signs of anxiety.** Your dog's first tell-tale signs of anxiety will most likely be calming signals such as yawning (Chapter 37). Respond to these by slowing down, pausing and adjusting your position. If the dog continues to show calming signals, give them a break. Leave them safely in their recovery crate or pen to calm down.
- **Use a calm approach.** Whatever you are doing, if your dog starts to look a little anxious, then give them more time, take a deep breath and slow your movements down. This will help avoid them getting really upset and trying to bite.
- **Muzzle your dog** whenever needed to keep yourself safe.

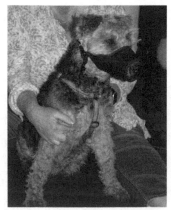

Using a muzzle

If you must get hands on with such an anxious dog, for example, to get them to the vet clinic, muzzle them for your own safety.

💡 **TIP:** *While your dog is muzzled, handle them gently, talk to them calmly, and give them enough time to accept what is happening. This will help them feel better and make them far more likely to cooperate with you next time.*

Figure 33: Take extra care to handle your dog gently while they are muzzled.

SECTION 7
Pain management

This section covers pain and how to deal with it.

CHAPTER 42
Is my dog in pain?

SUMMARY

BOX 1: SIGNS OF BACK OR NECK PAIN

- Yelping or squealing on being picked up or when trying to move
- Flinching during routine handling
- Not wanting to move much
- Trembling all over
- Rigid, hunched posture
- Excess panting, even if they are not too hot
- Licking or biting one area repeatedly
- Distressed facial expression: some dogs show the whites of their eyes, hold their ears tensely and look 'tight' across their forehead or around their eyes.

ASK YOUR VET'S advice if your dog shows any of these signs.

Many dogs are uncomfortable during a bout of IVDD, especially during the first few days or if there is a flare-up. Learn how to spot when your dog is in pain so that you can help them more easily.

Different dogs show pain in different ways. While a person with a sore back might moan and complain, dogs show less obvious signs of discomfort (see box 1).

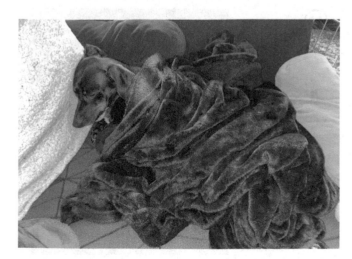

Figure 1: Some dogs don't want to move much when they are uncomfortable.

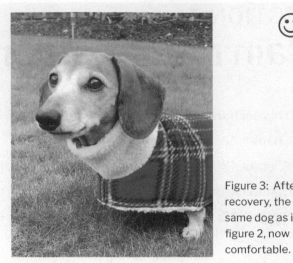

Figure 2: During a bout of pain, this dog trembled all over and had a tense expression on his face.

Lowered ears

Tight, bulging muscles around eyes

Lifting a front paw

Figure 3: After recovery, the same dog as in figure 2, now comfortable.

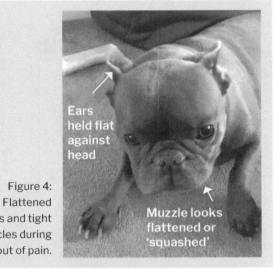

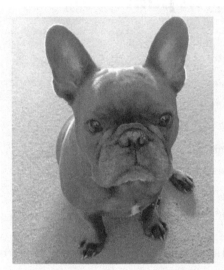

Ears held flat against head

Figure 4: Flattened ears and tight muscles during a bout of pain.

Muzzle looks flattened or 'squashed'

Figure 5: The same dog as in figure 4, now comfortable.

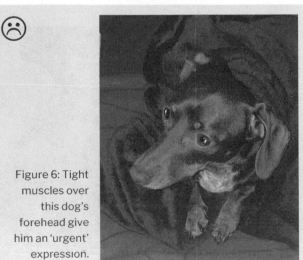

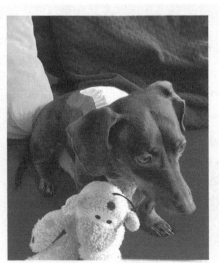

Figure 6: Tight muscles over this dog's forehead give him an 'urgent' expression.

Figure 7: The same dog as in figure 6, now comfortable.

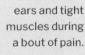
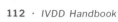

CHAPTER 43
Pain management – getting help from your vet

Your vet might prescribe one, two or even three different types of painkillers to be used together.

Most dogs become comfortable once painkillers have had time to take effect. But each dog responds differently. Your vet may need to reassess your dog and adjust the medication.

Once your dog is feeling better, remember to keep them safely confined to allow their body to heal (see Section 4, 'Your Dog's Recovery Area').

 CHECK WITH YOUR VET: Always ask your vet's advice before starting painkillers. They will select the correct dose and type depending on your dog's weight and medical history.

How to give medication

Follow the instructions on each packet regarding how often to give any medication, how much to give, whether it should be given with food, and whether it is safe to open capsules or crush tablets.

Most medications can be hidden in food (box 2). This works well for liquid painkiller, crushed tablets or the sprinkled contents of capsules. Stick with foods that your dog has done well with in the past. Check with your vet first: some capsules and tablets must be given whole, either by hand or by using a pill-giver (figure 9).

Let your vet know if you cannot give the medication. They may be able to prescribe something easier.

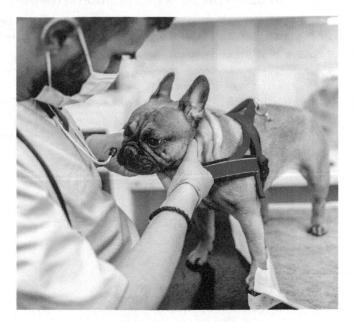

Figure 8: Your vet can assess your dog and prescribe painkillers.

BOX 2: HIDING MEDICATION IN FOOD

Try hiding their medication in:

- a spoonful of tinned dog food
- ham or sliced chicken breast
- a teaspoonful of liver treat paste or pâté
- a morsel of cheese.

⚠ **WATCH OUT** – cheese causes vomiting, runny stools or anal gland problems in many dogs.

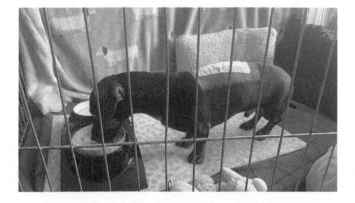

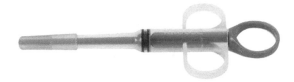

Figure 9: Medication can be hidden in food (a, left) or you could use a pill-giver (b, above).).

Types of painkiller

BOX 3: SOME MEDICINES PRESCRIBED FOR DOGS WITH BACK OR NECK PAIN

NAME OF MEDICATION	NOTES
NSAIDs (Non Steroidal Anti-inflammatory Drugs) Examples: Meloxicam (Metacam, Loxicom) Carprofen (Rimadyl, Carprodyl, Carprieve) Robenocoxib (Onsior)	NSAIDs reduce pain that is caused by inflammation. Follow the label instructions carefully. Most types of NSAID must be given with food or just after eating. Must never be used at the same time as prednisolone.
Gabapentin	Reduces 'neuropathic' pain (caused by damage to the spine or nerves). May cause slight sedation, especially at high doses.
Paracetamol	Reduces the dog's perception of pain.
Tramadol	Reduces the dog's perception of pain. Not effective in every dog. May cause slight sedation, especially at high doses.
Prednisolone	A steroid. Reduces inflammation. Often makes dogs hungrier and thirstier that usual. They may also pee more and pant a bit. Must never be used at the same time as NSAIDs.
Buprenorphine	An opiate painkiller. Usually causes obvious sedation.

🚫 **AVOID THIS: Never give your own supply of human medicine to your dog** unless your vet specifically tells you to do so. Some can be dangerous for dogs. Human preparations may also contain additives such as xylitol that can be harmful to dogs.

📞 **CHECK WITH YOUR VET:** Some medicines cannot be used together. Let your vet know if your dog is already taking anything else.

BOX 4: SIDE EFFECTS

A few dogs don't get on with certain medications.

📞 **ASK YOUR VET'S** advice if:

- your dog vomits or has runny or very dark coloured poo during treatment.
- your dog is unexpectedly lethargic or very restless. Some dogs behave differently when on certain painkillers.

CHAPTER 44
Caring for your dog during a pain episode

Dogs with back or neck pain sometimes yip or yelp unexpectedly, for example when lifted. Don't be too alarmed. They should start to feel better once their painkillers take effect. There is also plenty that you can do at home to help them.

Adjust your dog's activity regime

Set your dog up in a safe recovery area to help prevent pain flaring up. For a small dog, this is a crate or pen. For some larger breeds, a recovery room is needed.

Check that their crate or pen is large enough. Your dog will be more comfortable if they have enough space.

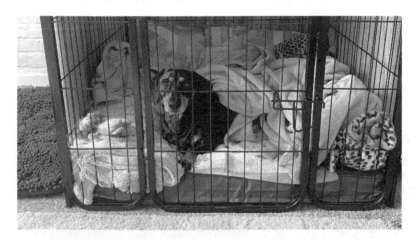

Whenever they are outside the crate, pen or recovery room, have your dog in your arms or under very close control on a harness and lead. Keep them on harness and lead whenever outdoors.

For more information, see

→ **Chapter 18 for advice on which size of pen or crate to use**

→ **Chapter 22 for a guide to comfortable bedding**

→ **Chapter 24 for advice on keeping them safe outside their recovery area**

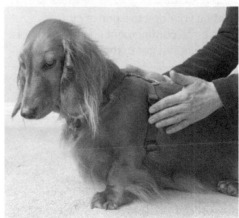

Figure 10 (above): Make your dog's recovery area comfortable. This will help them to feel more relaxed, so reducing the effects of any pain.

Figure 11 (left): Handle your dog gently to boost their confidence and allow their muscles to relax.

Handling your dog during IVDD recovery

✓ Take a deep breath and keep your own voice calm and reassuring when helping your dog.

✓ Use the top of their harness to steady them if they lose their balance or rush off.

✓ Use your hands and arms to 'contain' your dog as you lift and place them (Chapter 31).

CHAPTER 45
Help! My dog is on painkillers but is still in pain

Once your dog starts painkillers, it may take a few days for inflammation to settle down before they feel better. However, if they are very uncomfortable, getting worse, or not feeling better within a few days, speak to your vet. Doses may need adjusting, or they may need to add another medication.

Meanwhile:

❧ Check the table below for common causes of pain flare-ups. Adjust your dog's routine or home environment if needed.

❧ Handle your dog gently and calmly. For more details, see

→ **Chapter 37 for a guide to responding to their body language**

→ **Chapter 39 for some gentle handling techniques**

BOX 5: COMMON CAUSES OF PAIN FLARE-UPS

PROBLEM CAUSING PAIN FLARE-UPS	SOLUTION
Paws slipping on smooth or shiny flooring	Cover wood, laminate or tiled floors with non-slip matting (figure 11).
Hurrying across the floor to greet people	Confine your dog to a pen or crate. Once crate confinement ends, close doors so they cannot get to the front door.
Hurrying towards their food	Feed them in their crate or pen (figure 12).
Leaving the crate awkwardly over its lip	Lift your dog out carefully.
Moving over the doorstep to access the garden	Small dog: lift them over any steps. Large dog: use a harness and lead to slow your dog as they move over the doorstep.
Going off-lead in the garden	Keep your dog on the lead throughout the crate rest period. Introduce off-lead time gradually once they are ready.
Trying to jump	Confine your dog to a pen or crate. Once crate confinement ends, block off sofa access, or train them to use a sofa ramp.
Running or trotting too early	Use a lead to keep your dog very slow outdoors.
Turning tightly in a narrow crate	Switch to a larger, wider crate, or use a pen if your dog won't jump out.

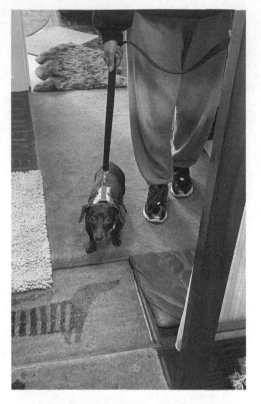

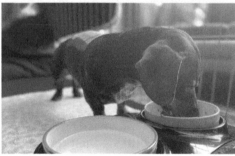

Figure 11 (top): Cover any slick flooring with non-slip mats.

Figure 12 (above): Feed your dog in their crate or pen.

SECTION 8
Toileting issues

CHAPTER 46
Toileting issues – what's happening?

Toileting can be a challenge for dogs during recovery from back or neck issues. The worst affected dogs cannot control their bladder or bowels at all. They need extra care and frequent clean-ups. Others have more control but may still have occasional pee and poo accidents indoors.

Mild problems

Occasional indoor 'accidents'
The change in routine can lead to toileting accidents indoors for some dogs. Those that have always used a certain spot outdoors or always walked a certain distance before 'doing their business' may take a while to adjust to their new routine. Others may pee or poo indoors because they cannot get outdoors in time.

Difficulty standing still for toileting
Dogs that are wobbly on their legs may find it hard to get into their usual squatting position, or to cock their leg to pee. This can happen to any dog recovering from a back or neck problem.

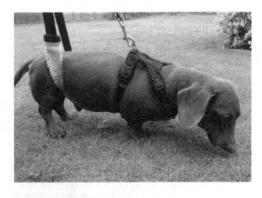

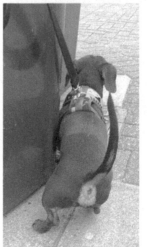

Figure 1 (above): Many dogs expect to go somewhere familiar outdoors as part of their natural toileting routine.

Figure 2 (left): It takes time to relearn how to stand and balance for toileting after a bout of IVDD.

Severe problems

Reduced bladder control

Urinary incontinence = A dog's inability to control when and where they pee

If your dog has more severe back or neck disease, the nerve supply to their bladder may be damaged. These dogs may want to pee but be unable to do so. And then, when it happens, they cannot control it. You might find patches or trails of pee indoors. Or lifting your dog may cause the pee to flow out – all over you! In these cases, the dog cannot control what is happening. It's not their fault.

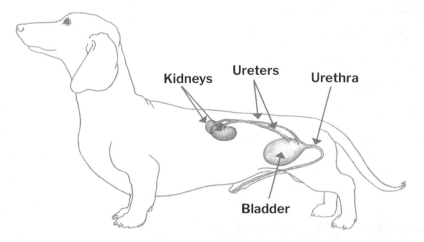

Kidneys Ureters Urethra Bladder

Figure 3: Diagram of the urinary system in a male dog. Urine is stored in the bladder. Dogs may be unable to control when or where they pee if the nerve supply to their bladder is damaged

---

BOX 1: TYPES OF URINARY INCONTINENCE

Different dogs have different issues with their bladder during recovery:

Unable to pee. The bladder gets very full. Now and again, some pee might overflow. If your vet asks you to express (squeeze out) your dog's bladder, it may feel firm and difficult to empty. This is called 'upper motor neuron bladder' and is often seen after injury to the middle of the back.

Weak, leaky bladder. The pee keeps leaking out, making these dogs difficult to keep clean. The bladder expresses easily. This is called 'lower motor neuron bladder' and is sometimes seen in dogs with lower back injuries.

The bladder can also become weak and leaky over time if it keeps overfilling. The wall of the bladder is eventually stretched and damaged if the dog cannot pee.

Reduced bowel control

Faecal incontinence (US: fecal incontinence) = A dog's inability to control when and where they poo

Some dogs with severe back or neck trouble cannot feel when they need to poo, or control when or where they do so. This is because the nerve supply to the bowel no longer works properly.

If poo seems to just drop out of your dog, or if they poo at any place or time and seem unaware that they are doing so, they have faecal incontinence.

CHAPTER 47
Helping your dog's toilet routine return to normal

A regular outdoor routine

Set your dog up for success by offering outdoor toilet breaks when they are most needed. This is likely to be first thing in the morning, last thing at night and after each meal. A regular routine, including outdoor toilet breaks, will help your dog relearn the good habit of peeing and pooing outdoors again.

SUMMARY

Whatever happens, be patient with your dog. It's not their fault. Telling them off will just make them anxious, and could lead to the problem getting worse.

✓ From the start, take your dog outdoors regularly for a chance to pee and poo.

✓ Praise them if they go in the right place. But don't scold them when they pee or poo indoors.

✓ Clean up any 'accidents' indoors promptly.

See Appendix 1 for suggested daily routines that you can adapt to your own dog's needs:

→ **use Routine 3, 'Leaky learners' if your dog is learning to walk and has poor bladder or bowel control**

→ **use Routine 6, 'Wheelers' if your dog is using wheels.**

From the start, carry your dog outdoors regularly and place them on the grass for a chance to pee and poo. If they seem reluctant, carry them to parts of the garden that they've used for toileting in the past. Use a harness and lead to keep them safe.

Until your dog can stand unsupported, they may find toileting very difficult. Whenever you take them outdoors, place them so that all four paws are flat on the ground and, if needed, use a sling to help them hold a standing position. Be patient – they may take much longer than normal to 'do their business'.

Learning to go in the right place

Once your dog either pees or poos in an appropriate place, immediately praise them: "Well done!". It's best not to scold them if they go indoors.

Clean up any indoor accidents promptly. Otherwise, your dog may start to think of that part of the house as their toilet! Until your dog's toilet routine is back on track, keep

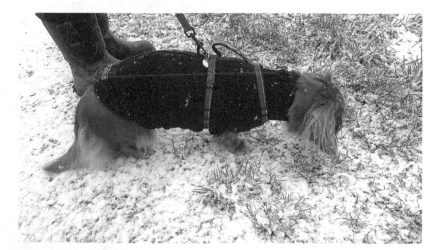

Figure 4: Take your dog outdoors at least every few hours during the day for toileting.

a 'pee & poo diary': make a note of what your dog passes and whether it's indoors or outdoors. If the problem does not resolve, show this to your vet and ask for advice.

CHAPTER 48

Caring for a dog with reduced bladder control

✓ **Clean your dog** and change their bedding when needed (Chapter 51).

✓ **Pee pads** (incontinence pads) are useful.

✓ **Take your dog outdoors** at least every few hours during the day to try and pee.

✓ **Limit the use of nappies/belly bands** until at least a few weeks into recovery (Chapter 52).

✓ **Encourage your dog to drink regularly.** Bring water to them if needed.

✓ **Contact your vet** if your dog does not pee within 12 hours (or 16 hours including overnight) and their bed is not wet.

✓ Your vet may ask you to express (empty) your dog's bladder (Chapter 49). Do this outdoors if possible.

Home care

There are cues outdoors to help your dog learn to pee normally again. These include the feel of grass against their paws, and being able to smell where they have been before. As your dog starts to recover, they might need to sniff the ground (to read their 'pee-mails'!) before they feel ready to pee. Keep them on the lead, but do let them sniff the ground.

→ see Chapter 28, 'Slings'

 TIP: Try putting some of your dog's pee onto a patch of ground outdoors. They will then know to use this place as a toilet area once their body is ready to do so.

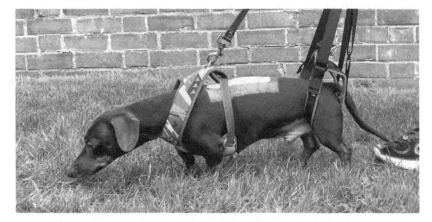

Figure 5 (above): For a boy dog, a wide sling would come too far forward and make it difficult for him to pee. Instead, use a narrow sling under his belly, or a hip lift sling as shown here.

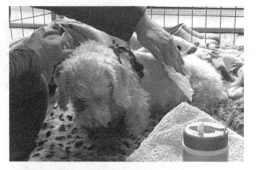

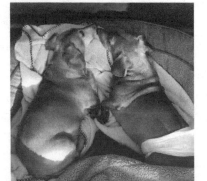

Figure 6 (above left): Clean your dog whenever needed (Chapter 51).

Figure 7 (above right): Pee pads are useful. Tuck them under the top layer of your dog's bedding (Chapter 22).

Figure 8 (left): The dog on the right is wearing a belly band. These can be very helpful for ongoing care. Don't rely on them though for at least the first few weeks into recovery (Chapter 52).

Getting help from the vet

ADVICE

Contact your vet for advice if:

🐾 Your dog does not pee within 12 hours (or 16 hours including overnight) and their bed is not wet – they may need urgent veterinary help.

🐾 Their pee has started to smell very strong.

Your vet can assess your dog and advise you. They might ask you to express (empty) your dog's bladder as part of the home routine (Chapter 49).

Bladder medication

Some dogs need medication to help their bladder work more normally. As with many medications, these are only prescribed when really needed, as there is a possibility of side effects (usually mild and temporary). Different treatments are chosen depending on your dog's general health and how their bladder is affected. Your vet or surgeon can advise you.

📞 **CHECK WITH YOUR VET:** Always ask your vet's advice before starting bladder medication. They will select the safe dose and type depending on your dog's weight and medical history.

Example treatment: For dogs with a firm bladder that is very difficult to express, prazosin (Hypovase) and diazepam (Valium) are sometimes prescribed together. These both come as tablets and are best given about 30-60 minutes before trying to express the dog's bladder.

Bladder infection (UTI)

During recovery from back disease, dogs are prone to getting a bladder infection, also called cystitis, a urinary tract infection or UTI for short.

A UTI is most likely within a few weeks of the initial injury or surgery and is often seen after a catheter has been used. UTIs can also happen months or even years later in any dog that still cannot pee normally.

If your dog's pee starts to smell very strong or looks cloudy, ask your vet to check for infection. They may need to prescribe antibiotics. Other possible signs of infection include more indoor 'accidents' than usual, drinking more than usual, and flinching when the bladder is expressed.

💡 **TIP:** *Be sure to give the whole course of antibiotics,* even if your dog starts to improve within the first few days. This reduces the risk of the problem coming back.

BOX 2: GETTING A URINE SAMPLE

To collect a urine sample, put a uripet (figure 12) or a clean container under you dog when they pee outside, or when you express their bladder. Bring the sample straight to the vet if you can – it's best tested within a couple of hours.

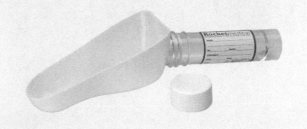

Figure 11: A uripet. Most vet clinics can supply these.

Urinary catheter

If your dog's bladder is too difficult to express, your vet may need to empty it by inserting a long tube (catheter).

Indwelling urinary catheter

This type of catheter is left in place for several days to allow the pee to flow out into a collection bag. Dogs are occasionally sent home with a catheter left in place, though this is quite unusual. More often, they are cared for in the hospital.

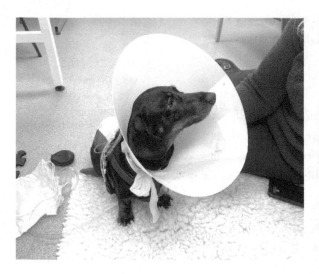
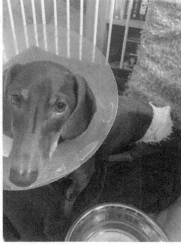

Figure 9 (far left): A dog with a urinary catheter during a clinic visit.

Figure 10 (left): At home, the catheter is covered with a layer of bandage wrap.

BOX 3: CARING FOR A DOG WITH A URINARY CATHETER AT HOME

Follow any instructions that you are given. You may be asked to check the catheter several times daily, perhaps to clean carefully around it, and either to drain urine from it or to empty the collection bag.

🐾 Take care not to pull the catheter out by mistake – some are easily dislodged.

🐾 Always wash your hands before and after doing anything with the catheter. Disposable gloves are also useful.

🐾 Don't let your dog lick at the catheter or pull it out. They should wear an Elizabethan collar (cone) if a catheter is in place.

🐾 Put your dog's water bowl within easy reach. Dogs do better if they keep hydrated.

 TIP: Use an Early Rest crate or pen, the smaller option, at least until the catheter has been removed (Chapter 18). If your dog drags themselves about too much, the catheter may get dislodged.

CHAPTER 49

Expressing your dog's bladder

Your vet may ask you to express (squeeze out) your dog's bladder two or three times a day until your dog can pee on their own. This prevents the bladder from overfilling. Otherwise, its wall could become permanently damaged by being stretched. Expressing the bladder also helps to keep bedding dry, and it reduces the chance of your dog getting a bladder infection.

Before you start

Give your dog a chance to pee naturally first. Carry them to a suitable patch of short grass outside, and let them stand or walk on a lead for up to a few minutes, with support from a hindquarter sling if needed.

Where to express your dog's bladder

The best place to express your dog's bladder is on the ground outdoors, with your dog supported in a standing position on soil, bark chips or short grass. Expressing the bladder outdoors will help your dog to associate peeing with being outdoors, so they can return to normal function more easily.

If there are times when getting outdoors is impossible, stand them on an incontinence pad, or have them rest or stand on a non-slip mat while you empty the bladder into a dish or onto some disposable padding.

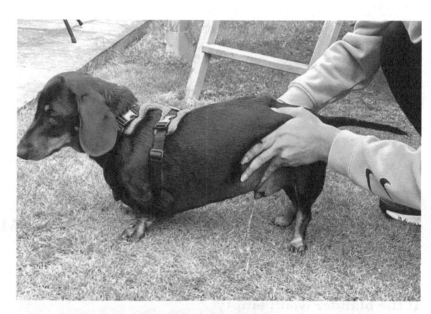

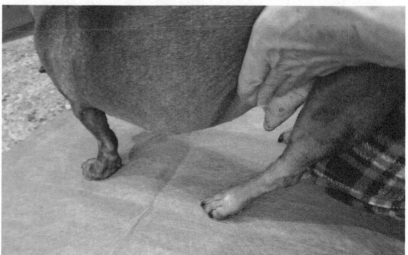

Figure 12 (top): Express your dog's bladder outdoors if possible.

Figure 13 (above): This dog is resting against his owner's knees while his bladder is expressed. For a female dog, keep yourself dry by crouching to one side of them instead.

How to express their bladder

1. **Positioning your dog.** Support them on all four paws in a standing position if possible. Or you can try with your dog lying relaxed on their side. Most people find it easier to use two hands to express their dog's bladder to start with, so have someone else in front to distract them.

2. **Using your hands.** Place your hands far back, one on each side of your dog's belly, and use the flat parts of your hands to apply slow, steady pressure to empty the bladder. Don't dig your fingertips in or try to overpower your dog.

3. **The last few drops.** Your dog's pee should come out in a steady stream when you express their bladder. Once this has stopped, let your dog relax for a moment, and then try again for another few seconds. There may be a few more drops to come out.

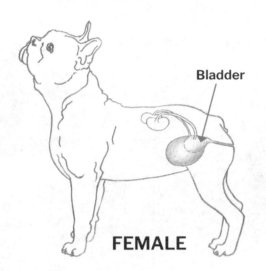
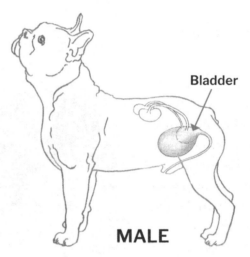

Bladder

FEMALE

Bladder

MALE

Figure 14: The bladder is far back in the belly, in the midline. It is smaller when empty (dashed lines) and expands forwards as it fills.

If the bladder won't empty

In some dogs, the bladder is full but it won't empty, even with quite firm pressure. Try taking your hands off, letting your dog relax for a moment, then trying again. You can also try with your dog in a different position, perhaps relaxed on their side.

If you still can't express your dog's bladder, ask your vet what to do. They might decide to prescribe medication to make it easier for the bladder to empty. Or they may need to pass a catheter into the bladder to empty it.

🚫 **BEST AVOIDED:** Don't dangle your dog over a drain, toilet or sink while expressing their bladder. A dangling position leaves them feeling helpless, may be unsafe for their spine, and won't help them learn to pee again.

CHAPTER 50

Caring for a dog with reduced bowel control

✓ Clean your dog and change their bedding when needed (Chapter 51).

✓ Take them outdoors for a toilet opportunity at least every few hours during the day.

✓ Check your dog's treats: don't give anything that makes their poos runny or sloppy.

✓ For long term incontinence, try cueing your dog to poo outdoors.

For many dogs, it takes a few days for the bowels to start working normally again after back or neck surgery or injury. Be patient, and take them outdoors several times daily for a chance to poo. If they have not passed anything within 5 days, let your vet know. In many cases, it can take even longer than this.

Dogs with severe back or neck problems may be unable to control when or where they poo. Give them plenty of outdoor toilet opportunities, keep them clean, and check that their diet is suitable (see below). It may also become possible to cue your dog to poo outdoors (box 6).

Diet for dogs with reduced bowel control

Some diets make the poos smaller, firmer and easier to clear away. Different dogs get on better with different diets. For many, sticking with their usual diet is the best option. If you do switch, make any diet change very gradually over at least a week to avoid a digestive upset.

- A very digestible complete dog food can help. Ask your vet's advice.

- Some owners find that feeding a complete raw diet makes the poos more manageable. Be particularly careful with hygiene when cleaning up after your dog if they eat raw food.

💡 **TIP:** *Avoid any 'extras' that might make their poos sloppy and difficult to clear away. For many dogs, this means avoiding cheese, milk, peanut butter, pâté and other rich foods.*

BOX 4: ADDING PUMPKIN TO THE DIET

Some owners find that adding a little cooked pumpkin to the diet makes it easier for their dog to poo.

To prepare: remove the seeds from fresh pumpkin or butternut squash, cut the flesh into chunks, and bake until soft before mixing it in with your dog's food. Or use canned pumpkin that contains no added sugar or other ingredients.

The dose: 1-3 teaspoonfuls per meal for a small dog, or 1-4 tablespoonfuls per meal for a large dog. Start with the lowest dose and increase gradually over a week if needed.

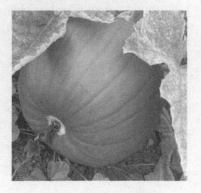

Coping with runny poo

Normal poos are log-shaped and easy to clear away. If your dog has runny poo (diarrhoea, or diarrhea in US), home care becomes more difficult as you must clean them and change their bedding more often.

Diarrhoea is very common after a sudden change of diet. Every dog is different, and some tend to have a slight bowel upset with certain foods. Too many treats can also cause this, as can rich foods such as cheese. Runny poo is also an occasional side effect of some medications.

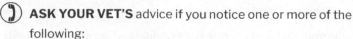

SAFETY ADVICE

**Box 5: Runny poo –
When to contact the vet**

☎ **ASK YOUR VET'S** advice if you notice one or more of the following:

- the poo is very watery
- your dog is refusing food
- there is any vomiting
- there is blood in the poo
- your dog does not seem right in themselves
- the problem started along with a new medication
- the poo does not start to get more solid over the first two days.

If in any doubt, ask your vet.

Diet during recovery

A simple, bland diet can help the poos firm up again. Many dogs do well with skinless, boneless chicken or white fish. Boil or microwave it until cooked through, then serve together with the same volume of rice. Or your vet may prescribe a special ready-made bland diet that is easy to digest. Stick strictly to the bland food, avoiding all treats and other extras until your dog's poos are back to normal. This may take a week or more.

In the meantime, check that your dog can reach their water bowl easily. They must drink regularly to keep hydrated. Keep an eye on them, and call the vet if needed (see box 5).

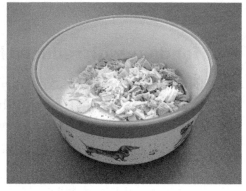

Figure 16: Chicken and rice .

BOX 6: LEARNING TO POO ON CUE

Outdoors, try triggering your dog to poo by tickling them under the tail, around the anus, or by holding an ice cube against this area. Many owners eventually find that this helps their dog do it in the right place at least once a day!

Different methods work for different dogs. Try using the following:

✓ a cotton bud.

✓ a disposable poo bag. Put it over your hand like a glove and tickle them with two or three fingertips.

✓ an ice cube – dip it in water to prevent freezer burn.

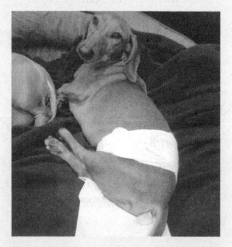

Figure 17: An ice cube placed under this dog's tail reliably prompted him to poo within one minute.

CHAPTER 51
Keeping your recovering dog clean

Clean and dry your recovering dog whenever needed. This will help prevent skin sores and leave them feeling better about the situation.

Check your dog's coat and remove any traces of pee or poo after each 'accident' and after expressing their bladder.

✓ Use unscented baby wipes for small clean-ups.

✓ If your dog is very wet or dirty, sponge-bathe them carefully (box 7).

✗ Don't try to give them a proper bath or shower during recovery. They could wriggle or slip and reinjure themselves.

To help keep your dog clean and comfortable, check and change their bedding and pee pads frequently. (See Chapter 22, 'Your dog's bedding')

Avoid dry shampoos. Though they may mask any smell, they don't remove dirt properly from the coat and can cause skin irritation.

Apply a barrier cream to protect areas that keep getting wet or dirty. Barrier creams can only be used on clean, dry skin, and are best reserved for areas that don't have much hair such as under the tail. Your vet may recommend one, or use a human nappy cream such as Sudacrem on unbroken skin.

 TIP: *Old towels are handy both for mop-ups and for tucking under a leaky dog whenever you need to lift them.*

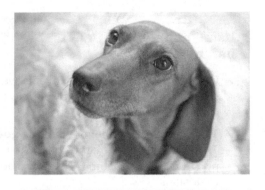

BOX 7: HOW TO SPONGE-BATHE YOUR DOG

1. Wash your hands before and after cleaning your dog, and/or wear disposable gloves.

2. Rest your dog on a pee pad, old towel or, with care, on the lawn.

3. Use an old towel, cloth or kitchen paper to wipe most of the contamination from your dog's coat.

4. Clean affected skin using plenty of water. Dilution is the solution to pollution! Use a sponge, together with water either in a bowl or spray-bottle.

5. Towel dry your dog gently, taking care not to knock them off-balance. Pay special attention to any skin folds, finishing off with a paper towel if needed.

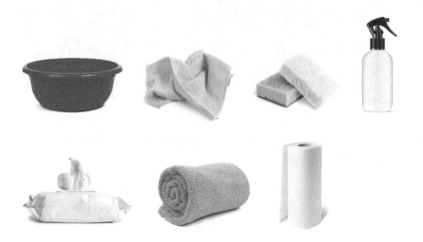

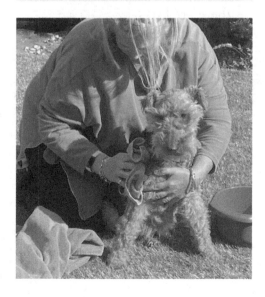

Figure 18: Sponge-bathing a dog.

CHAPTER 52

Nappies (diapers) and belly bands

Using nappies and belly bands

✓ **Change them frequently.** Never leave your dog sitting in a wet or dirty nappy or belly band as this can cause skin sores.

✓ **Take them off whenever your dog goes outside.** This will give your dog the chance to pee and poo normally. Also, the fresh air will be good for their skin.

✗ **Don't have your dog rely on nappies or belly bands too early.** During the first few weeks of recovery, it could slow down their return to normal toileting behaviour.

Nappies (diapers in the US) and belly bands can help to keep your home clean if your dog is incontinent. However, they have a few drawbacks. Firstly, dogs that rely on nappies or belly bands during the first few weeks of recovery may find it more difficult to learn to pee and poo outdoors normally. Secondly, dogs easily get skin sores under a nappy or belly band, especially one that is left on for too long. Their skin is therefore best left uncovered at least overnight, and whenever possible outdoors.

Belly bands

A belly band is a piece of elasticated fabric that wraps around the dog's midriff. They are for male dogs only and are used to catch pee (but not poo).

✓ They come in various sizes. Measure your dog carefully and follow the manufacturer's size guidelines.

✓ Line the band with something absorbent. Buy purpose-made liners or use sanitary towels. Change the liner or towel whenever your dog pees.

✓ Buy at least one spare belly band. You will need to wash it now and again if there are leaks.

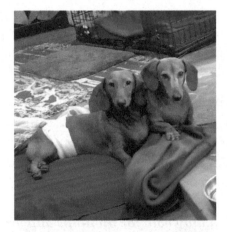

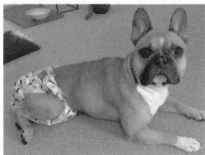

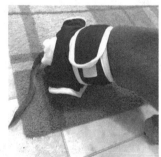

Figure 19 (top left): A belly band can help keep your home clean. Leave it off when possible to allow air to reach your dog's skin.

Figure 20 (below left): This 13 kg (29 pound) dog is wearing a size 5 human disposable nappy with a reusable dog nappy over the top.

Figure 21 (below right): A dog nappy with a tail hole.

Nappies (Diapers)

Special disposable or washable nappies can be bought in various sizes for male or female dogs, with or without a hole for the tail. Human nappies can also be used, and you can cut a hole for the tail if needed.

Though designed to catch both pee and poo, their usefulness is limited. Leaks can be a problem, especially for male dogs, and for long-bodied breeds such as dachshunds. If your furry friend poos in a nappy and then moves about, this may leave you with an unpleasant clean-up job!

Some owners report that the human nappies are most absorbent, but that they slip off easily. Keep them in place by putting either a Velcro-fastening reusable dog nappy, or human swim pants, over the top.

CHAPTER 53
Will my dog learn to pee and poo normally again?

The good news is that most dogs do recover the ability to pee and poo normally, usually around the time that they start to walk again.

Once your dog has regained control of their bladder, continue to be patient with them. After a major bout of back disease, some are left needing to pee more often than before, and you may find that they do so with excitement when you return home.

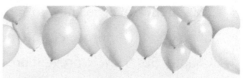

During recovery, your dog's first outdoor pee and poo(p) can each be cause for celebration!

A few dogs are unfortunately left unable to control when or where they pee or poo. This is more likely in the following situations:

1. **Paralysed dogs.** Dogs that have lost all function of their hind legs, especially if they have also lost deep pain sensation (see box 9).

2. **Severe lower back problems.** Dogs with lower back injuries (within the L4 to S3 section of the spine) have slightly less chance of regaining bladder or bowel control than dogs with neck or mid-back injuries.

3. **Pugs with 'constrictive myelopathy'**, a gradual onset back issue. Many of these dogs are left incontinent despite still being able to walk.

Even if very poor bladder or bowel control turn out to be long term issues, many owners eventually find a home routine that works well.

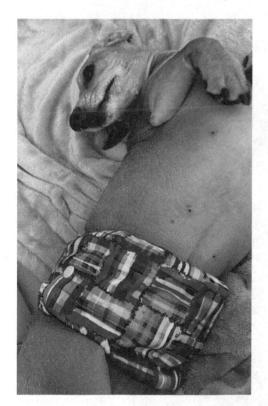

Figure 22: Dogs can enjoy a good quality of life even if their toileting has not returned to normal

BOX 9: TOILETING — CHANCES OF RECOVERY FOR GRADE 5 DOGS

Dogs that have lost their deep pain sensation are very severely affected and may be left with reduced bladder and bowel control in the long term (see Appendix 3, 'Clinical grade chart').

🐾 Unfortunately, dogs that do not regain deep pain sensation within the first 6 weeks after injury or surgery are very unlikely to pee or poo normally again.

🐾 Of those that do regain deep pain sensation, around 4 out of 10 dogs are left with unreliable bladder or bowel control. They might dribble pee indoors now and again, or they may poo indoors at times, either because they cannot get out in time or because they are not aware of needing to go.

SECTION 9
Skin, paws and claws

This section explains how to care for your dog's skin, paws and claws during recovery.

Chapter 54:   How to keep your dog's skin healthy

Chapter 55:   How to prevent pressure sores

Chapter 56:   Paw problems

CHAPTER 54

How to keep your dog's skin healthy

Skin easily gets damaged if dogs drag themselves about. Dogs with poor bladder or bowel control are prone to skin irritation due to soiling. Skin damage can also be caused by lying in one position for too long.

Take special care of your dog's skin during recovery.

Checking for skin damage

Check your dog's skin at least twice a day, paying special attention to the areas shown in figure 1. Watch for areas of:

* patchy hair loss
* pink or red skin
* thickened skin

Let your vet know if you find any damaged areas. They are more treatable if caught early.

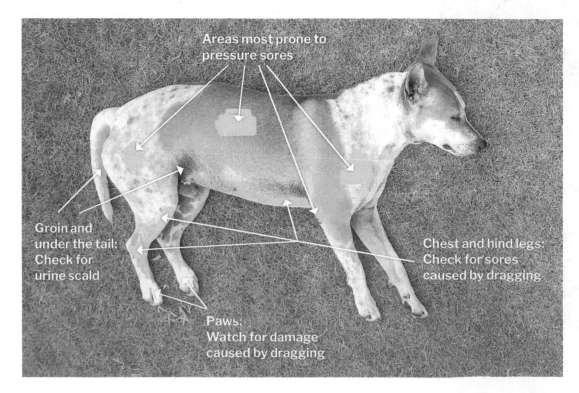

Areas most prone to pressure sores

Groin and under the tail: Check for urine scald

Paws: Watch for damage caused by dragging

Chest and hind legs: Check for sores caused by dragging

Figure 1: Parts of the body most often affected by sores and other skin damage

Preventing problems

Sores can take a much longer time to heal than we expect. It's best to take steps to prevent them from happening in the first place (see box 1).

BOX 1: HOW TO PREVENT SKIN PROBLEMS

PROBLEM	AREAS AFFECTED	HOW TO PREVENT THIS
Sores due to soiling with pee or poo (urine scald)	Groin Under the tail	**If your dog has poor bladder or bowel control:** ✓ clean and dry them regularly ✓ have fur clipped short in the groin region and under the tail – it will make it easier to keep the skin clean and dry ✓ after drying, apply a barrier cream such as Sudacrem. ✗ don't leave a nappy (diaper) on all day → See Section 8, 'Toileting issues'
Pressure sores (bed sores)	Bony areas such as the elbows, side of ribcage and hip bones	✓ Provide soft, clean bedding ✓ Keep your dog clean & dry ✓ Turn your dog regularly if needed → See Chapter 55
Grazes, sores and claw damage caused by dragging	Skin at the top and sides of paws Claws may be worn down too short	Don't let your dog drag their paws, especially over concrete. 1. **Until they can walk:** Support them with a sling for walking. Confine them to a pen, crate, or small carpeted room. 2. **If they can walk but are wobbly:** Keep your dog slow using harness and lead. Keep walks brief - they'll drag their paws more once tired. Walk on grass, not concrete. 3. **Long term problems:** Consider using boots in addition to the above advice. → See Chapter 56

Caring for sore skin

First aid for sore skin involves gentle sponge-bathing and drying (Chapter 51). If the skin is not broken, apply a barrier cream such as Sudacrem.

See box 1 to check what might have caused the problem. Adjust your dog's home care as needed. For example, you may need to provide better bedding, or prevent your dog from walking on concrete.

Contact your vet if any skin is red, puffy or broken, or if milder signs don't start to improve within two days of home care. Sores can flare up quickly so ask your vet's advice straight away if in any doubt.

 TIP: *If the sore is under a nappy, leave the nappy off for as much of the day as possible. Most skin sores heal better if left uncovered.*

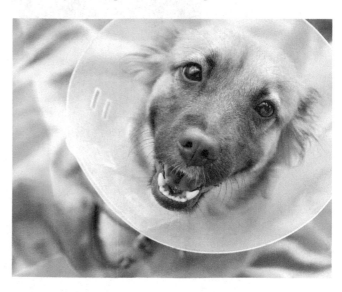

Figure 2: Don't let your dog chew a sore area. They may need to wear an Elizabethan collar.

CHAPTER 55

How to prevent pressure sores

Lying in one position for too long can lead to pressure sores (bed sores). Skin is more easily damaged and infected if left dirty, so dogs with poor bladder or bowel control are more prone to problems.

Preventing pressure sores   **TOP TIPS**

✓ Provide soft, absorbent, padded bedding (Chapter 22).

✓ Clean your dog's skin by sponge bathing as often as needed, then dry carefully (Chapter 49). This is particularly important if they have poor bladder or bowel control.

✓ Change their bedding as soon as it is wet or soiled.

✓ If your dog cannot change their position without help, turn them at least every four hours during the day.

Turning your dog

Must all dogs be turned?

No, turning is only essential for dogs that cannot change their position without help. This includes dogs that cannot use any of their legs, and those that cannot lift their head. Most dogs that can move about a bit by themselves do not need turning, even if unable to walk. Ask your vet's advice.

BOX 3: POSITIONING YOUR DOG

1. Lying on their right side

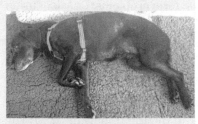

2. Lying on their left side

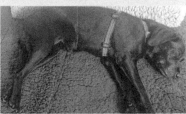

3. Lying on their front (sphinx position)

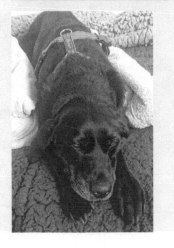

When?

If needed, turn your dog at least every four hours during the day. Fit this in with their toilet breaks, home exercises or bedding changes. If your dog is considered particularly prone to bed sores, then your vet may also advise you to turn them every few hours through the night.

How?

Turning your dog involves placing them in a different position every time you return them to their bed. Plan which way round to position your dog before lowering them to floor level.

Position your dog on their front to eat, drink and interact with people. If they are too weak to prop themselves in this position, support them carefully with bolster cushions, rolled blankets or towels.

💡 **TIP:** *Remind yourself by keeping a note of when you last turned your dog and which way they were lying.*

CHAPTER 56
Paw problems

Preventing paw problems

Box 4: To help prevent paw problems

✓ **Use a lead** to slow your dog down (see Chapter 29, 'Using the lead). This will help them to step properly instead of dragging.

✓ **Keep walks short**. Rest your dog in a pushchair if needed. Dogs drag their paws more once their legs are tired.

✓ **Support your dog with a sling** if they cannot walk. Lift the sling just as much as is needed to prevent the paws from scraping along the ground. Take special care to lift the sling if your dog moves over concrete or stony ground.

Paws are easily grazed and claws worn down if they drag over hard ground. If your dog tends to put their paws upside-down or to drag their feet, follow the advice in box 4 to help keep their feet healthy.

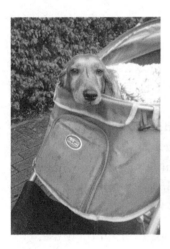

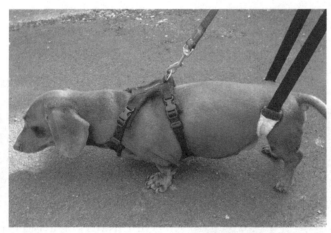

Figure 4 (far left): Rest your dog in a pushchair before they get too tired.

Figure 5 (left): If your dog cannot walk, support them with a sling, and use the lead to slow down their front end.

Checking for sore feet

Check your dog's paws at least once a day for for bald patches, grazes, pink sore areas, and damage to the tips and sides of the claws.

If their claws are wearing down fast, take extra care to follow the advice in box 4. The sensitive 'quick' inside the claw could become exposed if they get too short.

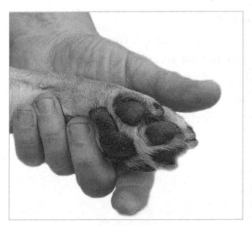

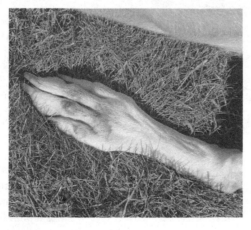

Figure 6 (far left): A healthy paw.

Figure 7 (left): Hair loss and pink patches caused by knuckling the paws when walking.

Caring for sore feet

Follow the advice in box 5 to allow the skin to heal.

> ### Box 5: Allowing sore paws to heal   **TOP TIPS**
>
> ✓ Avoid all hard ground:
>   - ✓ Carry your dog over concrete or stones
>   - ✓ Only let them walk on soft ground such as grass.
> ✓ Keep walks short. A pushchair can be very useful.
> ✓ Boots may also be needed while the skin heals.

> ### BOX 6: SALT WATER
>
> Mix 1 teaspoon of salt* into one cup (225ml; 8 fluid oz) of water.
>
> *Use non-iodized table salt.*

Clean grazes or sores with water or salt water (see box 6), and pat dry with tissues or a clean towel. If the skin is not broken, you can apply Sudacrem or a barrier cream recommended by your vet.

Contact your vet if skin on your dog's paws is broken, red, puffy or oozing.

Boots

Boots can be useful in the following situations:

- ❧ To protect damaged paws while they heal
- ❧ Ongoing paw protection for dogs that are not expected to walk normally again.

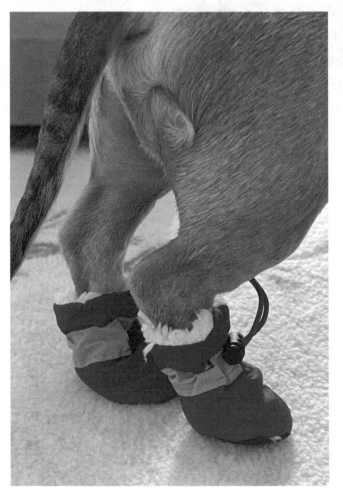

The drawback of using boots

Dogs may be less likely to learn to walk while wearing boots. This is because they can no longer feel where they are placing their feet, so they tend to step less carefully.

For this reason, avoid boots, or limit their use, while your dog is learning to walk. Instead, restrict your dog to soft areas, matting and carpet indoors, and walk them slowly and carefully when outdoors. Lift them if needed over hard ground, or use a sling, harness and lead to prevent their paws from dragging.

Choosing boots

Boots should be easy to get on and off, and they should fit snugly but without pinching or cutting off the circulation. If they wear through too fast, Shoe Goo (shoe repair glue) applied to their soles can extend their lifetime.

Figure 8: Lined soft fabric boots with a simple tie-cord design are suitable for smaller breeds.

SECTION 10
Home exercises

Section 10 includes exercises that can be used at home during recovery.

Posture exercises:

Lead exercises:

Ask your physiotherapist to assess your dog and help get you started if needed.

CHAPTER 57
Getting started with posture exercises

> **TOP TIPS**
>
> ✓ **Practice makes perfect.** Repeat an exercise through the week to help your dog learn.
> ✓ **Keep learning sessions short.** Muscles tire very quickly in dogs with IVDD.
> ✓ **Keep it positive.** Handle your dog gently and use small rewards during training.
>
> Learning to walk is a big challenge. Exercises break this down into small chunks that your dog can manage.

Posture exercises involve helping your dog to get into safe, natural positions:

* Stand
* Sit
* Sphinx position (lying on their front)

Over time, dogs get stronger through practising these postures and movements. Being helped from one position to another reminds them how to move in a natural way.

These are particularly useful exercises for dogs that cannot walk. Your dog should gradually learn to move with less support from you. Their nervous system can even rewire itself during the recovery process, forming new connections that help your dog to get up and walk.

Each dog learns and recovers at a different rate. For a tailored programme of exercises to suit your dog's current ability, ask for referral to a physiotherapist.

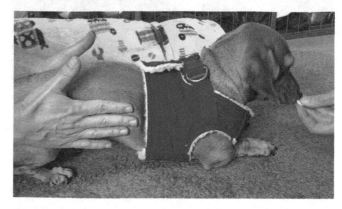

Figure 1: Set aside some of your dog's food to use as rewards during exercise sessions.

Which exercises should I include?

Start with standing practice (see Chapter 58).

Once you and your dog are confident with standing practice, you can gradually start to add in the exercises from Chapter 59. Don't add more than two new exercises per week.

Each dog is different, and some find certain exercises too challenging. If an exercise is not working as described, or if your dog objects to an exercise, miss it out or ask a physiotherapist for advice.

Safety

Use a harness
It's surprising how fast a dog can move, even if they cannot walk! Fit your dog with a harness. Its top acts as a useful grab-handle in case they're about to fall or scramble away.

> **SAFETY ADVICE**
>
> **Box 1: Safety for exercises**
>
> ✓ Only do exercises on non-slip footing.
> ✓ Put a harness on your dog – it's a useful grab-handle
> ✓ Do exercises at floor level.
> ✓ Keep a close eye on your dog. Don't let them fall or try to dash off.

Where to do exercises
Exercises are best done on the floor or, with good control, on the lawn. Only consider using a raised surface if you cannot get down to floor level. You must always keep your dog safe. Carpet, short grass or rubber-backed matting are perfect surfaces for exercises.

If you must use a raised surface like a table, take special care. Cover it with non-slip matting for better grip. Don't take your eyes off your dog, even for a moment. They must wear a harness.

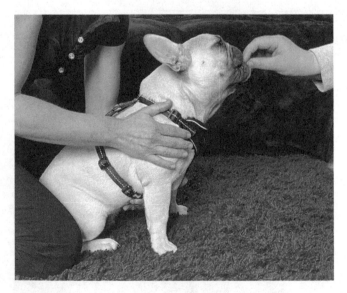

Figure 2: Exercises are often easier with two people.

How many people are needed?
One person can usually manage on their own with a smaller dog at floor level. However, exercises are often easier with two people, one to position the dog, and the other to keep them focused.

It's more difficult to help larger breeds with exercises. For a weak large dog, two or even three people may need to work together. Ask your physiotherapist for advice.

CHAPTER 58
Standing practice

What is standing practice?

Help your dog hold a standing position on non-slip flooring. This strengthens muscles and helps them learn how to stand again. Most dogs learn to stand before they can walk.

Support your dog on all four paws for ten seconds, then lower them gently to the floor.

When to start

Standing practice can start within the first week after injury or surgery in most dogs. Start with just 10 seconds of supported standing twice a day. Check with your vet or physiotherapist if you are not sure, and always follow the safety guidelines (see box 1).

BOX 2: STANDING PRACTICE

- ✓ Help your dog stand on all four paws with support from your hands.
- ✓ Only attempt this on non-slip footing.
- ✓ Position yourself behind your dog.
- ✓ Your dog should face forward (see box 3).
- ✓ Check that each paw is the correct way up.
- ✓ Lower your dog gently to the floor before they tire. Don't let them fall.

Instructions

1. **Help your dog up.** With your dog facing some food, position yourself behind their tail. Lift them gently to their feet using a hand under their belly or between their hind legs. Steady them with your other hand if needed.

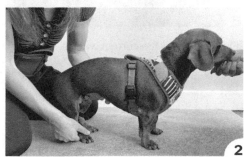

2. **Correct their paw position.** Check that each paw is the right way up. To correct the position of a hind paw:
   a) Keep a hand under their belly for support.
   b) Lift the paw with your thumb on top of the toes.
   c) Replace the paw the correct way up (pads touching the floor).
   d) Pause for two seconds with your thumb on top of the paw.

   Work methodically, correcting one paw and then the other. Be patient.

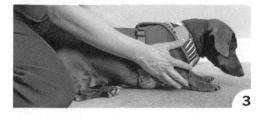

   Keep standing. Give as much support from your hands as needed. Keep your dog standing briefly – just ten seconds on day one.

3. **Lower your dog gently down to the floor.**

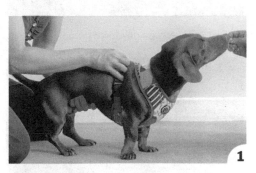

Tips for standing practice

Here are three ways to keep your dog facing forwards during the exercise:

a) Ask a friend to **distract them from in front** using food or a toy.

b) **Smear food onto a lick mat** and attach it vertically at their head height.

c) **Do the exercise at mealtimes.** Your dog will focus on their bowl of food.

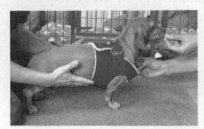
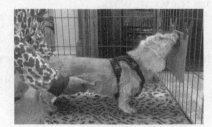
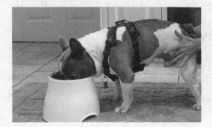

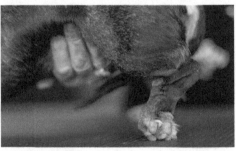

Figure 5: A paw upside-down (knuckled).

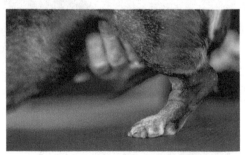

Figure 6: A paw the correct way up.

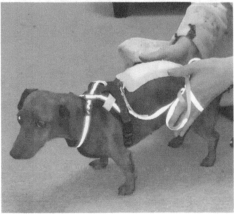

Figure 7: A dog standing straight.

Checking their position

Dogs with IVDD sometimes stand with their legs crossed, with one leg out to the side, or with a paw upside-down. They don't always know where their legs are.

During standing practice, correct your dog's position so that they stand straight on all four paws:

✓ Each paw should be the correct way up (figure 6).

✓ They should have 'a leg at each corner' (figure 7).

 TIP: *Always support your dog under their belly while correcting their paw position.*

In severe neck disease, all four legs may be weak. In that case, support your dog under both their chest and rear end.

For a small dog, spread your fingers wide to support under their chest. You can also use rolled towels or cushions to help prop your dog. A larger dog with severe neck disease may need three people for support.

Building up standing practice

If your dog's hindquarters are very weak, you will need to support their full weight. It may feel as if you are doing all the work, like holding up a puppet. Stick at it nevertheless. As you repeat the exercise over the following days and weeks, they will eventually need less support.

Standing for longer
Start standing practice twice daily, making the first attempt just ten seconds of supported standing. Once familiar with the exercise, build it up gradually to a minute at a time.

Reducing your support
If your dog can hold some of their own weight, gradually reduce the strength of your support. Don't let them fall!

Helping your dog stand straight
With practice, you may find that you can support your dog with hands on either side of their hindquarters. This will help you keep their body straight. If they sway to the right or left, nudge or coax them very gently back to the centre.

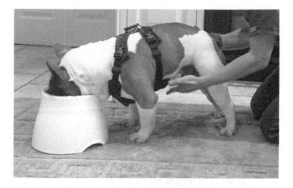

Figure 8: As your dog learns to stand, hover your hand just under their belly in case their legs give way.

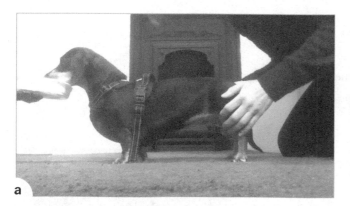

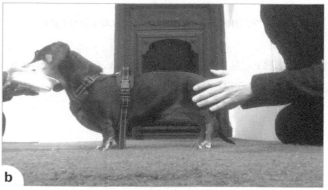

a   b

Figure 9: A hand on each side of the hindquarters can provide firm support (a) or very light support (b).

Keep checking their paw position. Each hind paw should be under each hip. Each paw should be the correct way up.

→ **Once you are confident with standing practice, see Chapter 59, 'Further posture exercises'.**

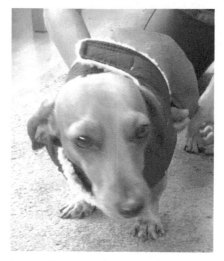

Figure 10: Support with a hand under their belly while correcting their paw position with your other hand.

CHAPTER 59

Further posture exercises

Once you and your dog are comfortable doing standing practice (Chapter 58), add in further exercises one by one. Don't overdo it! Add no more than two new exercises per week. For a programme tailored to your dog's needs, ask for referral to a physiotherapist.

Posture exercises　　**TOP TIPS**

✓ Avoid fatigue: keep exercise sessions brief.

✓ Handle your dog gently during exercises.

✓ Reward them as soon as they get something right. Use a morsel of food, say "well done", or let them play with a favourite toy.

✓ If your dog is getting tired, cut the session short (see box 6).

BOX 6: SIGNS OF TIRING

❧ Knuckling their paws upside-down more often than before

❧ Becoming less steady on their feet

❧ Muscle tremor in the hind legs

❧ Your dog becoming less cooperative as the exercise continues.

Once you and your dog are confident with several posture exercises, start to link them into a sequence. Keep it simple to start with. Focus on quality rather than quantity. It's better to do one exercise well than to do several exercises badly.

→ **See Appendix 5 for advice on combining exercises**

⚠ **CHECK FIRST** with your vet before starting these exercises if your dog has joint disease or a leg injury such as a broken bone.

Exercise 1: Hind paw sequencing

Hind paw sequencing moves the main joints of each hind leg and helps retrain a stepping action.

When to start?
Get confident at standing practice before trying hind paw sequencing.

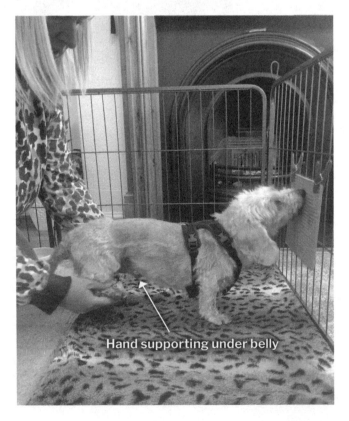

Hand supporting under belly

Figure 11: Lift and place a hind paw while supporting your dog with your free hand.

Instructions

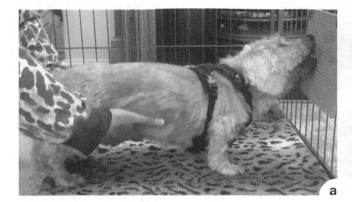
a

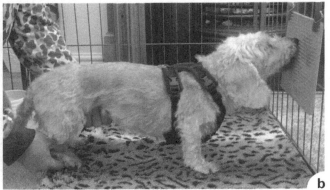
b

Start with your dog in a balanced standing position (see Chapter 58). Support them with a hand under their belly.

Slowly and deliberately lift and place a hind paw so that it steps on the spot.

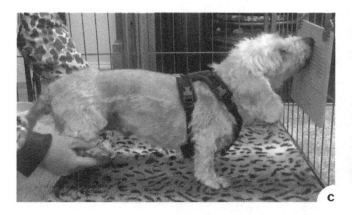
c

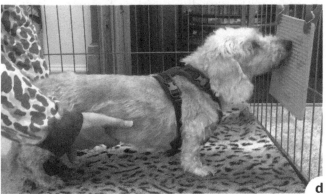
d

TIP: *Place your thumb on top of the paw whenever you lift a leg.*

Switch hands, then lift and place the other hind paw.

TAKE CARE! Don't let your dog fall: support them as needed with your free hand as you lift each paw.

BOX 7: PAW SEQUENCING – A BASIC WORKOUT

Try the following once daily:

1. Standing practice (Chapter 58)
2. Lift and place right paw
3. Lift and place left paw
4. Repeat steps 2 and 3
5. Lower your dog gently to the floor for a rest.

Optional: add an extra step each day until they are doing 4 steps with each hind paw.

Don't overdo this exercise. It encourages some dogs to lean too heavily on their front paws. Check with your physiotherapist if needed.

→ **See Appendix 5 for advice on combining this with other exercises.**

Exercise 2: Small backward weight shift

The small backward weight shift improves hindquarter strength and balance. It also reminds dogs with weak hind legs not to lean too heavily on their front legs.

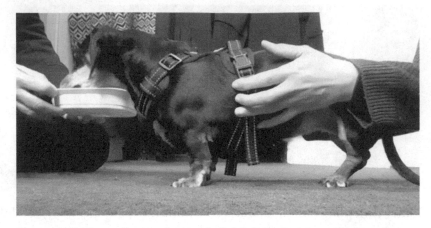

Figure 13: Shift your dog's weight back slightly from their harness. It's a tiny, gentle movement.

When to start

Only start this once your dog can stand for at least five seconds without support. You and your dog must first be confident with standing practice (see Chapter 58).

Instructions

1. Start with your dog standing facing forward on non-slip footing. To keep them focused, they could be eating from a raised food bowl, or using a lick mat fixed at head height.

2. Check that your dog's paws are the correct way up and that they are standing straight. Correct if needed (Chapter 58).

3. Tuck your middle fingers into the side pieces of the harness. Gently and slowly, use your fingers to coax your dog's bodyweight back by just 2-4 mm (1/8th of an inch)

4. Keep them in the new position for three seconds, then release the backward pressure.

5. Repeat once or twice more.

⚠ **TAKE CARE!** Don't let your dog fall: support them as needed with your free hand if you need to lift a paw.

Exercise 3: Stand to sit

Help your dog into a balanced sitting position. Stand to sit frees up their hind leg joints, strengthens muscles, and helps them relearn how to sit. When sitting correctly, dogs fold their hind legs into a tight zigzag, with paw pads touching the floor ready to push up to stand (see figure 14a).

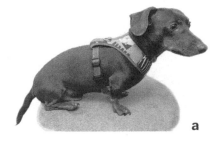 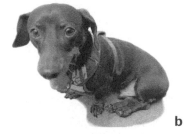 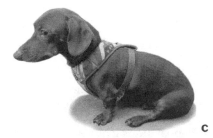

Figure 14: (a) A neat sit with hind legs folded. (b) A crooked sit with both hind legs off to one side. (c) A straight sit, but with the hind legs too straight and the tail tucked under.

When to start

Start stand to sit once you and your dog are confident with standing practice (chapter 58).

Instructions

┌───┐

Stand to sit   **SUMMARY**

✓ Work together with a helper if possible. Small food rewards are useful.

✓ Start with your dog standing supported on non-slip footing (see Chapter 58, standing practice).

✓ Lower their bottom gently to the floor.

✓ Keep their haunches straight as they lower into the sit.

✓ For the best sit, help your dog fold each leg into a neat zigzag (see box 9).

└───┘

Work with a friend to turn this exercise into a positive game. Your dog gets a reward each time they sit. Position your friend in front of the dog with a few food morsels. Meanwhile, stay behind your dog to support their weight and correct their position.

1. **Start with your dog standing straight on non-slip footing.** Check that each paw is the correct way up.

   When ready, ask the dog to sit: Have your friend prompt the dog by saying "Sit!" while motioning slightly upward with a treat-holding hand.

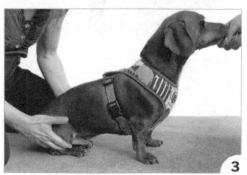

2. **Help them lower to a sit:** Your dog might try to sit if they know the command. If not, use a hand on each side of their rear end to help them lower gently to the floor. Give them a food reward as soon as their bottom touches the floor.

   💡 **TIP:** *Help them stay straight:* While lowering to a sit, your dog's rear end might start to flop to one side. Use a hand on each side to keep them central.

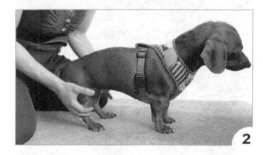

3. **Help them hold the sit position:** With a hand on each side, prop your dog so they don't flop to the right or left. Keep each hind leg folded in a zigzag. If your dog's rump rolls backwards, use your knees as a backstop.

   To help keep your dog sitting, have your helper hold food or a toy directly in front of the dog's nose so they can lick at it. If food is too far away from your dog's face, they might try to scramble forward.

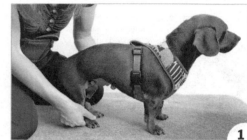

   Lower your dog gently to the floor for a rest.

BOX 9: PRO TIP

Help your dog fold their hind legs into a zigzag (a) as they sit. Use a finger just in front of their hock (b) to help a leg to fold if needed.

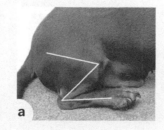
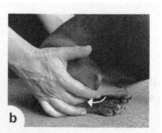

Exercise 4: Sit to stand

Sit to stand strengthens the dog's hindquarters and teaches them to push up off the floor. Start this once you are confident with standing practice (see Chapter 58) and Exercise 3, stand to sit.

> **Help your dog get up from a sitting to a standing position.**

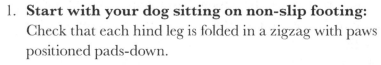

SUMMARY

Sit to stand

✓ Work together with a helper if possible. Small food rewards are useful.

✓ Start with your dog sitting supported on non-slip footing (see Exercise 3, stand to sit).

✓ Use your cupped hands or fingertips under their seat bones to help them up.

✓ If they are very floppy, support instead with a hand or arm under their belly.

✓ Keep all four paws on the floor. Don't lift their rear end too high.

✓ Neaten their standing position if needed.

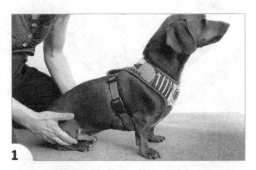
1

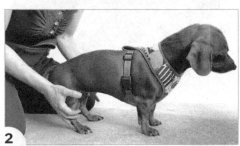
2

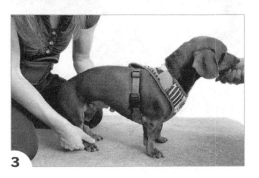
3

Instructions

Work with a friend to turn this exercise into a game. Your dog gets a reward each time they sit, and another each time they stand.

Position your friend in front of the dog with a few food morsels. Meanwhile, keep yourself behind your dog to support their weight and correct their position.

1. **Start with your dog sitting on non-slip footing:** Check that each hind leg is folded in a zigzag with paws positioned pads-down.

   When ready, ask the dog to stand: Have your friend prompt the dog by saying "Stand!" or "Up!"

2. **Help your dog up:** Use cupped hands or fingertips under their seat bones to help them rise. If your dog is very floppy, lift with a hand under their belly. Your dog should get the food reward as soon as they are standing.

   💡 **TIP:** *Don't lift their hindquarters too high.* The paw pads should stay on the floor.

3. **Neaten their standing position:** Check that your dog is standing straight, with a leg at each corner and each paw the correct way up (see Chapter 58, standing practice).

LIFTING FROM UNDER THEIR SEAT BONES

There are two seat bones, one on each side under the tail.

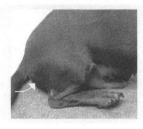

→ See Appendix 5 for advice on combining sit to stand with other exercises.

Exercise 5: Slow head turn

This exercise improves balance and core strength. Help your dog hold a stable standing or sitting position while they turn their head to each side.

When to start

Start the slow head turn in a standing position once your dog can stand supported for at least 10 seconds (see Chapter 58).

Start the slow head turn in a sitting position only once your dog can sit for at least 10 seconds with their legs folded into a zigzag, with your support (see Exercise 3, stand to sit).

Instructions

1. Start with your dog either standing or sitting. From behind, support them as needed in this position.

2. Position a helper in front of the dog with a small container of wet food held just in front of the dog's nose. Allow the dog to lick at the food.

3. The helper should move the food very slowly to their right side, then back to centre, then to the left side, and back to centre. Allow the dog to lick at or get bits of food as they move their head.

4. From behind, correct the dog's position and support their weight as needed. Can they hold a steady stand or sit position while moving their head?

5. Repeat once or twice. Finish the exercise with your dog's head pointing straight ahead.

 TIP: *Do this exercise very slowly for best effect.*

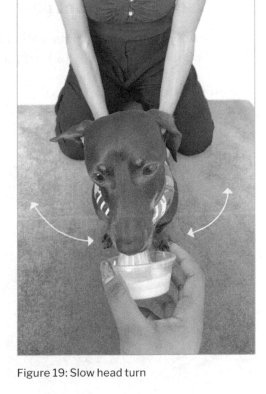

Figure 19: Slow head turn

FOR THE SLOW HEAD TURN, TWO PEOPLE WORK TOGETHER

Person 1: helps the dog to stay in a standing or sitting position.

Person 2: uses food to encourage the dog to look slowly to the right and to the left side.

Try using an old yoghurt pot containing a smear of wet dog food, mashed boiled carrot, or liver paste.

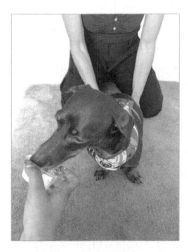
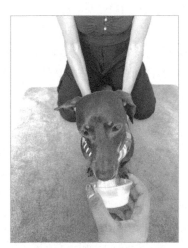
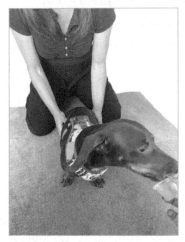

Exercise 6: Lift a front paw

This exercise improves strength and balance. It's mainly enjoyed by dogs who already know how to lift a paw on command.

> **Help your dog hold their sitting position as they lift a front paw.**

When to start
Only start 'Lift a front paw' once your dog can sit straight for at least 30 seconds (see Exercise 3, stand to sit).

Instructions
Work with a helper. Position them in front of the dog with tiny pieces of food such as crumbs of chicken hidden in their hand.

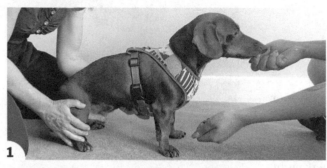

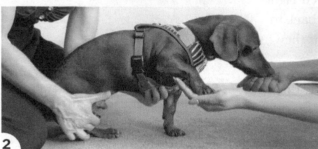

1. **Start with your dog sitting.**

   With a hand on each side, prop your dog from behind so they don't flop to the right or left. Aim to keep each hind leg folded in a zigzag. Use your knees as a backstop, if needed, to prevent the dog's rump from rolling backwards.

2. Have your friend **prompt the dog to lift a front paw. They say "Paw!".** As soon as the dog lifts a paw, they get a food reward. From behind, support your dog under their chest to give them more confidence to balance on three legs.

   Repeat with the other paw.

Tips
✓ **Help your dog hold a stable sitting position** while they lift each paw. From behind, use your hands if needed to prevent the haunches from rotating to one side and to keep the hind legs folded into a zigzag.

✓ **Practice both sides equally.** For many dogs, one paw is easier to lift than the other.

✓ **Give extra support** with a hand under their chest, if needed, as they lift the more difficult paw.

✓ **Don't let your dog lean** their raised front paw heavily on a hand. That would be cheating! Instead, when they touch a hand with their paw, keep that hand 'light' and move it about slightly.

Building it up

More reps
If your dog enjoys this exercise and manages it easily then repeat morning and evening. Add one rep each week until they are lifting each paw three times. Do less if your dog is getting tired.

Lift a paw for longer
If they manage well then gradually encourage them to hold each paw up for longer. Increase this very gradually, up to a maximum of 10 seconds per paw. For example, your dog may be able to hold each paw up for 1 to 2 seconds longer each week.

Exercise 7: Sit to sphinx

Sit to sphinx reminds the dog how to lie down in a straight, coordinated way. The sphinx position is also useful for dogs learning to push themselves up off the floor. It's the easiest lying position from which to get up.

Help your dog down into a neat, symmetrical lying position.

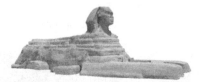

Figure 22: The Great Sphinx of Giza

When to start

Only start sit to sphinx once you and your dog are confident with standing practice (Chapter 58) and Exercise 3, stand to sit. Your dog will find this exercise easier if they already know the "Down!" command. If your dog dislikes being put into a down position, miss this exercise out or ask your physiotherapist for advice.

Instructions

Position a helper in front of the dog with a few food morsels. Meanwhile, stay behind your dog to support their weight and correct their position.

1. **Start with your dog sitting on non-slip footing.** Check that they are straight. Each hind leg should be folded in a zigzag with paws positioned pads-down (see Exercise 3, stand to sit).

   Prop your dog's rear end with your hands and/or knees to keep it still and stable.

2. **When ready, ask your helper to tell the dog to lie down.** They should put a treat at floor level and say "Down!".

3. **Help your dog lie down.** Some IVDD dogs will go down unaided. Otherwise you can 'walk' their front legs down:
   a) Support under their chest with one hand (see box 11).
   b) Use your other hand to lift and step a front leg forward. Swap hands and repeat with the other front leg.
   c) At each step, bring your dog's chest lower to the floor and say "Down!".

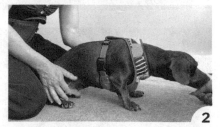

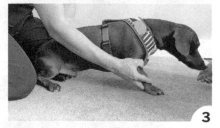

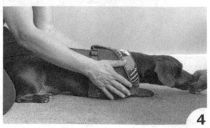

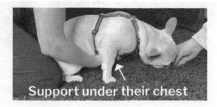

4. Allow your dog to get the **food reward** as soon as their chest touches the floor.

   Neaten their lying position from behind: They should be lying straight like a sphinx. Use a hand on either side to straighten them if needed. Check and correct their hind legs: each should be folded in a zigzag with paws positioned pads-down. As you correct your dog's position, have your helper distract them with food from directly in front.

BOX 11: TIPS FOR SIT TO SPHINX

✓ **Support under their chest** with one hand, if needed, as they go down.
✓ **To help keep your dog in the sphinx position**, position the food centrally so that they can lick at it. If food is too far away, they might scramble forward. If food is held off to one side, they will not lie straight.

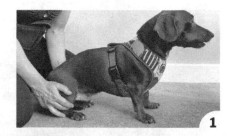

Support under their chest

Exercise 8: Sphinx to sit

Sphinx to sit improves coordination and core strength. Together with sit to stand, this exercise helps your dog learn how to get up off the floor.

Help your dog rise to a straight sitting position.

When to start
Start this exercise once your dog is confident with Exercise 7, sit to sphinx.

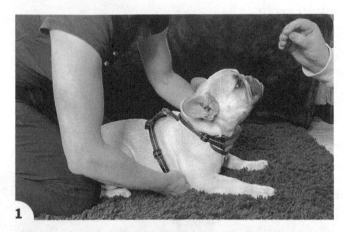

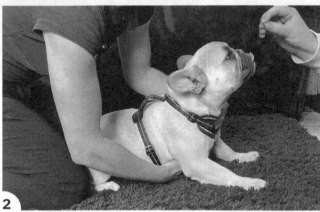

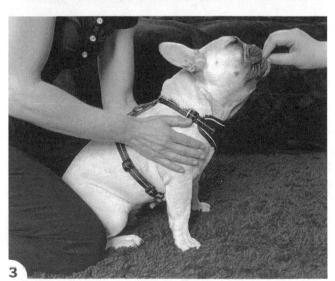

Instructions

1. **Start with your dog lying on their front on non-slip footing.** Check that their body is straight. Each hind leg should be folded in a zigzag with paws positioned pads-down. Correct if needed. Use your hands and/or knees to help keep your dog's rear end steady throughout this exercise.

2. **When ready, ask the dog to sit.** Have a helper prompt the dog up to a sit by raising a treat to sitting level and saying "Sit!". Don't give them the treat until they are sitting.

   Help your dog up to a sitting position. While you keep their hindquarters steady, your dog might be able to get up to a sit. If not, use on-off pressure from a hand under their chest to coax them up.

3. Your dog should get the **food reward** as soon as they are sitting.

   Neaten their sitting position: Check that your dog is sitting straight. Their hind legs should be folded in a zigzag with paws positioned pads-down. Correct if needed. As you correct your dog's position, have a helper distract them with food from directly in front.

CHAPTER 60
Getting started with lead exercises

Equipment needed

Dogs do best with exercises that fit in naturally with their daily routine. The most useful ones tend to look the least impressive! You will just need the following equipment:

* ❧ A good harness (Chapter 26)
* ❧ A fixed-length lead (Chapter 27)
* ❧ For dogs that cannot walk, a sling (Chapter 28)

Why do lead exercises?

These exercises strengthen the hind legs, improve coordination and prompt dogs to lean less heavily on their front legs.

Lead exercises help dogs to become steadier on their feet.

When to start lead exercises

Each dog has different needs. Follow your vet's advice as to how long your dog can be on their feet, how fast they can go, and when they can start using a step, kerb or ramp.

For more advice on when to add each exercise, see

→ **Chapter 10 if your dog can walk**

→ **Chapter 14 if your dog cannot walk**

BOX 12: WHICH EXERCISES TO USE

If your dog is using a sling: use the starter exercises in Chapter 61.

For dogs that can walk without a sling: start with the exercises in Chapter 61. Once your dog is steadier on their feet, gradually add exercises from Chapter 62.

📞 **Check first with your vet** before allowing your dog to trot, or to step over a doorstep.

First check your lead technique

Have your dog on harness and lead for all the exercises in this section. You will need to hold the lead as follows for the exercises to work:

* ✓ **With sling support:** Hold the lead in one hand and the sling in the other hand (figure 25). See Chapter 30 'Using the sling'.

* ✓ **Without sling support:** Hold the lead in two hands (figure 26). Always keep the lead pointing back from its clip. Have your thumb on top of the lead. Walk very slowly. See Chapter 29, 'Using the lead'.

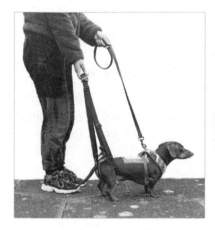

Figure 25: Hold the lead in one hand, and the sling in the other hand.

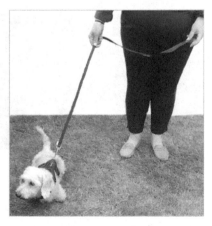

Figure 26: Walking a dog without a sling. It's best to hold the lead with two hands.

CHAPTER 61

Starter lead exercises

Exercise 1: Three, two, one, stop

Lead exercises help dogs to become steadier on their feet.

Why?

To strengthen the hind legs and make them more stable.

✓ During sling walking, this exercise encourages dogs to use their hind legs.

✓ It is also useful for dogs with weak or wobbly hindquarters, and for those that still knuckle their paws occasionally.

When to start

Use three, two, one, stop during outdoor toilet breaks. It's safe to start this exercise during the first week following injury or surgery, even if your dog is using a sling. Continue it throughout recovery until your dog can walk, trot and run normally.

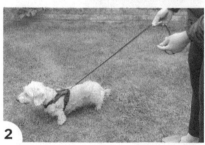

1

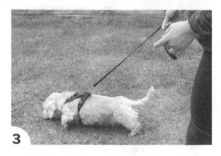

2

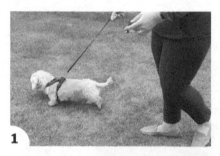

3

Instructions

Start by walking with your dog on a harness and lead. Walk on their weaker side if they have one.

1. **Slowing to a stop.** Gradually ask your dog to stop, using fingertip pressure on the lead. Give them at least a count of three to come to a standstill.
2. **The stop.** Have your dog stand still for just a moment.
3. **The start.** Let your dog start walking again. For tips on getting your dog started, see box 14.

How often?

Start by doing 'Three, two, one, stop' twice daily. Build up gradually over the next few weeks, for example by adding an extra repetition every third day.

BOX 13: CHOOSING WHEN TO STOP

Do this exercise:

🐾 when your dog is moving forward enthusiastically.

🐾 when they were not about to stop anyway. For example, stop them as they cross the lawn towards their favourite sniff-spot.

BOX 14: TIPS FOR GETTING YOUR DOG TO START WALKING

✓ They might start walking if you release the pressure on the lead slightly.

✓ Try saying "Come on, let's go!".

✓ For dogs that don't need a sling, try prompting them to go by pointing forward with the hand furthest from your dog.

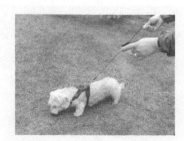

Exercise 2: Mats track

Why?

Textured mats improve the dog's paw position sense ('proprioception'). Mats also offer a grippy, safe surface on which to try some first steps.

When to start

'Mats track' is safe to start early, even when the dog is still being sling-walked. Start it once your dog is allowed on their feet for long enough to make it part of a toilet break. This exercise is useful throughout recovery.

Instructions

Setting it up

1. Place a straight line of non-slip mats to create a pathway for your dog.

2. Lay the mats from the crate or pen to the garden door.

3. Include mats with at least two different textures. For example:

   - yoga mat
   - coir doormat
   - rubber-backed fluffy bathmat
   - non-slip rug

Walking over the mats

Walk your dog slowly on harness and lead over the line of mats. As your dog walks, keep the lead pointing backwards from its clip to encourage them to step slowly and carefully.

 TIP: *Walk them in their preferred direction – towards the garden if they love to go outdoors, or back to the crate or pen if they long to get back there. Your dog will use their legs better if they are enthusiastic.*

 REMEMBER: If the route indoors or out includes a doorstep, lift your dog over it until your vet is happy for them to step over.

Walk your dog slowly over a line of textured mats on their way in or out of the house.

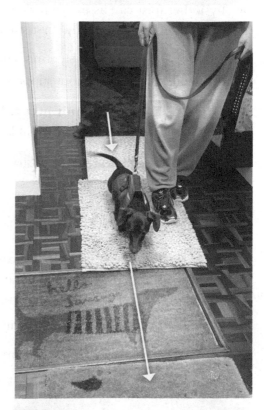

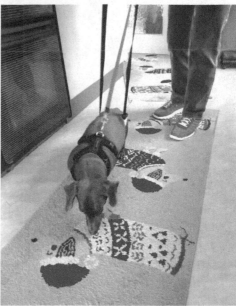

Figure 29 (top): Walking slowly over a mats track.

Figure 30 (above): 'Mats track' is suitable for dogs that use a sling. This dog is following a food trail.

Learning to walk without a sling

When to start walking without a sling

Most dogs eventually learn to walk without a sling. Each dog recovers at a different rate. Your vet or physiotherapist can assess your dog and advise you on when to start reducing sling support. As a general guide, you can try the first stage of the process when:

✓ your dog makes regular step movements with each hind leg during sling walking

✓ and they can stand without support for at least a few seconds.

⚠ **TAKE CARE: Don't just take the sling away!** Follow stages 1-4 of the process below. Wait for your dog to be comfortable and confident with each stage before progressing to the next one.

If your dog struggles with this, restart standard sling-walking and leave the transition process until they are stronger.

Instructions

Stage 1: Lower the sling while standing

a) Lower the sling now and again when your dog stops to stand. While lowering the sling, slow your dog from the lead so they cannot rush ahead.

Watch your dog: can they stand without sling support?

b) As your dog moves off, raise the sling again to give as much support as needed.

Repeat this exercise at each sling-walk attempt.

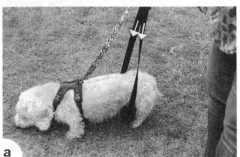 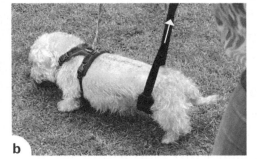

Figure 31: a. The sling being lowered while the dog is standing. b. The sling being raised as the dog starts to walk.

Stage 2: Lower the sling briefly while walking

Your dog is ready for this once they can stand without much wobble with the sling lowered. Now try keeping it lowered briefly as they start to walk off again. Raise the sling if your dog needs more support.

 TIP: *Set this up so that your dog is very motivated to walk (perhaps towards food, a favourite person, or back towards the house). At the same time, slow their front end down using the lead and harness.*

Walk on your dog's weaker side if they have one.

Repeat stage 2 each time you take your dog outdoors. Eventually, you will hardly need to use the sling at all while your dog is walking slowly. They are then ready for stage 3.

Stage 3: Walk two metres (6 feet) without the sling

Before you start

Your dog is ready for this once they can manage Stage 2 easily. They should be able to walk or stand, without risk of falling, whenever you lower their sling (see Stage 2).

You will need a fixed length lead at least 160 cm (73 in) long.

→ **See Chapter 29, 'Using the lead'.**

Setting it up

Use a piece of level ground. Lawn is ideal, or use a line of non-slip matting indoors. Have your dog walk towards food, or put one of their favourite people on the 'finish line' so they can walk towards them. Clip a lead to the top of your dog's harness.

Walking without a sling

Aim for your dog to walk just 2 metres (6 to 7 feet).

1. **Position your dog.** Use two hands to place them gently on the 'start line' in a standing position. If they are excited, steady them from the top of their harness so that they don't rush forward before you are ready.

2. **Position yourself next to or just behind your dog's tail.** Stand on the side of your dog's weaker hind leg if they have one. Hold the lead with two hands (Figure 32)

3. **Steady your dog from the lead as they walk.** As your dog moves off, walk very slowly so you don't get ahead of them. Always keep the lead pointing back from its clip (Figure 33). Slow your dog from the lead, especially if they are rushing or if their steps are wobbly.

Repeating the exercise

If your dog manages this exercise but looks wobbly, repeat it once a day until they are stronger. Continue to use the sling for their remaining outdoor time, lowering the sling now and again as in stages 1 and 2. Once your dog can stay on their feet reliably, they can progress to stage 4.

Steady your dog as they take their first steps. Use a harness and fixed length lead.

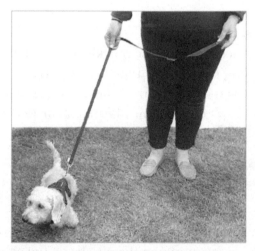

Figure 32 (left): Hold the lead with two hands.

Figure 33 (below): Aways keep the lead pointing back from its clip.

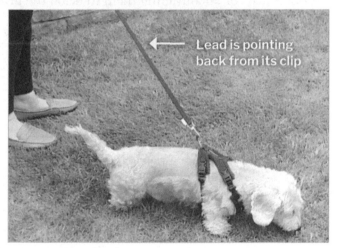

← Lead is pointing back from its clip

Stage 4: Build up walking on the lead without the sling

Once your dog can walk at least two metres with their paws the correct way up, try them on the lead without the sling for part of each outdoor toilet break.

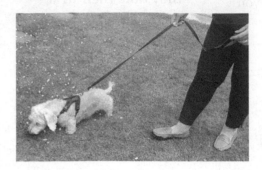

Figure 34: Walking on the lead without the sling.

Starting to walk without a sling

✓ Walk slowly, using the lead to keep your dog slow.

✓ Stop and stand still when your dog chooses to stop.

✓ Always keep the lead pointing back from its clip (see Figure 33).

✓ Walk on the side of your dog's weaker hind leg.

✓ Keep walking sessions very short.

How long to walk

Your dog's muscles will fatigue quickly. Let them walk without the sling for no more than 60 seconds at a time to start with, even if they seem enthusiastic. Over the next few days to weeks, you may be able to increase this gradually to 5 minutes depending on how they get on.

Watch for signs of tiring (see box 15). Give your dog a rest if you notice any of these, even if their walking time is not yet up.

BOX 15: SIGNS OF TIRING

🐾 Footfalls becoming less neat and regular.

🐾 A leg starting to buckle or give way.

🐾 Paws placed upside down (knuckled).

🐾 Legs crossing when placed.

You can rest your dog by picking them up, putting them into a dog pushchair, bringing them back indoors early, or encouraging them to lie on the grass next to you if the weather is fine.

→ See Chapter 70 for advice on increasing your dog's walk length.

CHAPTER 63
Further lead exercises

Add these in very gradually once your dog can walk without a sling.

→ **See Chapter 60, 'Getting started with lead exercises' for more information,**

Exercise 1: Varying the lead pressure

Why?
To strengthen and coordinate their hind legs and core muscles.

When to start
Start this exercise once your dog can stop and start on their walks without stumbling or falling.

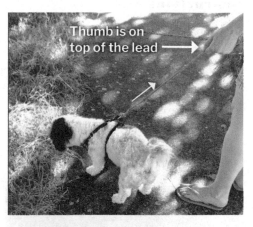

Instructions
1. **Pick the right moment.** Try this when your dog has chosen to stop for a while, for example to sniff at their favourite spot.
2. **Position yourself.** Stand slightly behind and to one side of your dog. Hold the lead with two hands. The hand nearest to the dog should have its thumb pointing down the top of the lead towards them (see figure 35).
3. **Vary the lead pressure.** Apply very gentle pressure through the lead so that it goes just taut, hold for 1-3 seconds, then slowly release the tension. Repeat.

The lead should slowly go taut as pressure is applied, then go slightly slack as it's released.

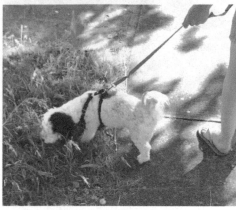

Troubleshooting
During this exercise, if your dog steps backwards or sits down, your lead pressure was either too sudden or too strong. Try again next time more slowly and gently. If it's not working, leave this exercise until your dog is stronger.

Figure 35a (top): Applying gentle backward pressure through the lead.

Figure 35b (above): Your dog should be comfortable to stand and sniff about while you vary the lead pressure.

Building it up
Start by varying the lead pressure for up to 10 seconds per walk. If you dog is happy and can stand securely during this exercise, build it up gradually week by week. This is a useful exercise to continue for many months, even after full recovery.

 TIP: *Stand mainly on your dog's weaker side* if one of their hind legs is weaker than the other. This exercise will help to get that leg stronger.

Exercise 2: Stepping over a hosepipe

Why?

Stepping over a hosepipe improves coordination and proprioception (paw position sense).

When to start

Start this exercise once your dog can walk with fairly regular steps and without knuckling their paws. Fit it in with your dog's routine. It could be done as often as once daily or just once a week.

Instructions

Setting it up

Before bringing your dog outside, drop a flexible garden hosepipe onto the lawn or patio so that it forms a few random loops. Adjust it if needed so that each loop lies flat on the ground.

This exercise is best done slowly. Your dog should walk, not trot, over the hosepipe.

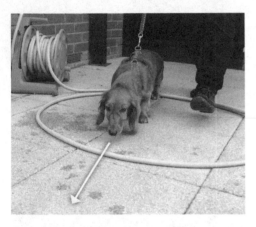

Figure 36: Keep the lead pointing backwards as your dog steps over the hosepipe.

The exercise

Walk your dog on harness and lead across the lawn in a straight line over the hosepipe. Like a child stepping over pavement cracks, dogs tend to step in the gaps between the hosepipe loops. Walk slowly, keeping the lead pointing backwards to encourage your dog to step carefully.

 TIP: *Stop before your dog is tired.* Once or twice over the hosepipe is usually enough.

Variations

This becomes a slightly different exercise each time because the hosepipe loops fall randomly. As an optional extra, add in one or two plastic hula hoops for your dog to step over.

Exercise 3: Trot for a count of five

Why?

✓ This is a safe, gradual way to get dogs trotting again. Up until this point, during early recovery, your dog should go no faster than their walking pace.

✓ Later in recovery, trotting for just five seconds is a useful coordination exercise.

When to start

Before trying trotting, your dog must walk well, without knuckling, crossing or dragging their paws. Some dogs trot as soon as they're allowed to move faster, and they find it easy. Many others take months to relearn how to trot, particularly after a severe back injury.

 IMPORTANT: Only let your dog go faster than their walk speed once your vet or surgeon is happy for them to do so.

What is a trot?

The trot is a regular, bouncy movement in which the paws touch down in diagonal pairs. Dogs have three main paces:

1. Walking: Their slowest pace
2. Trotting: A little faster. Healthy small breed dogs mainly trot when they 'go for a walk'.

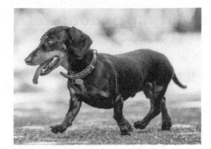

Figure 37a: A dog trotting.

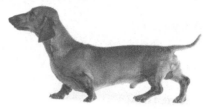

Figure 37b: A dog walking.

3. Running: A bounding movement that is faster than trotting.

Most healthy dachshunds, French bulldogs and other small breeds trot at the same speed as their owner's fairly slow walk.

Instructions

a) Trot on level ground, with good footing. Path or mown grass are suitable. Pick a moment when your dog is walking on the lead, and they are keen to move faster.

b) Allow them to go slightly faster for a count of five seconds

c) Use the lead to slow them to a walk again.

Try this just once per walk to start with.

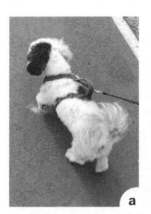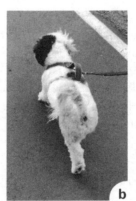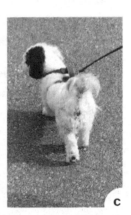

💡 **REMEMBER:** *Keep the lead pointing backwards from its clip throughout,* even when you want your dog to go faster. This will help them to stay balanced.

BOX 16: TIPS FOR TROTTING

✓ Walk next to your dog, don't run. If you move too fast, your dog will need to run to keep up with you.

✓ If they need encouragement, say "Come on, let's go!", and put a little bounce in your step.

✓ Only try a few seconds of trot at a time.

Building up the trotting

Only increase the trotting once your dog manages it easily. At first, many dogs 'cheat' by running, bunny-hopping, or pacing instead. Ask a friend to video your dog's gait and show this to your vet or physiotherapist.

Increase their trotting bit by bit:

1. Gradually build up the length of time trotting. Once they are allowed to trot, start with five seconds of trotting at a time. If they manage this easily, add an extra second every other day.

2. Once your vet or physiotherapist is happy for you to do so, start to increase the number of times per walk that your dog trots.

3. Build up gradually over weeks or months until your dog is trotting for at least half of each walk. Always slow them to a walk for downhill slopes, bumpy ground, kerbs and other obstacles.

⚠️ **TAKE CARE: Don't trot** if your dog is having a bad day or a flare-up. Just walk them slowly.

Exercise 4: Stepping over a ramp or doorstep

Why?

This helps to prepare your dog for returning to a normal lifestyle. It also improves their coordination and proprioception (paw position sense).

When to start

Only walk your dog over a doorstep or ramp once your vet is happy for you to do so. This depends on your dog's current walking ability, the length of their legs and the height of the step. With care, shallow ramps can be used for some dogs within the first few weeks of recovery. Most dogs should wait longer than this before using the doorstep.

Instructions

Setting it up

You might first need to make your garden step shallower, fit grip tape to your door threshold or fit a ramp (Chapter 74). Check that there is enough room for you to walk next to your dog through the doorway. Place a large non-slip mat by the door if your floor is slippery.

Going over the ramp or step

Walk your dog slowly on harness and lead over the step or ramp. Keep the lead pointing backwards from the clip throughout to encourage your dog to step carefully, one paw at a time. If you let them go too fast, they might bunny-hop, slip or scramble.

How often?

Fit this in with your dog's routine, starting to use the step or ramp for access indoors and outdoors.

 TIP: If your dog needs motivating, have someone call them from in front, or lay a food trail.

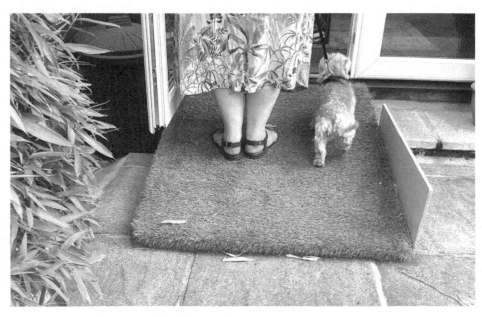

Figure 39: Walking slowly over a ramp.

Home massage and touch techniques

> Section 11 covers home massage, range of movement, and other touch techniques.
>
> Chapter 64: Introduction to touch techniques
> Chapter 65: Home massage
> Chapter 66: Range of movement
> Chapter 67: Sensory touch work
> Chapter 68: Pinch withdrawal exercise

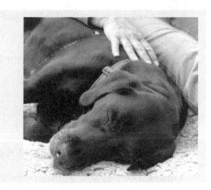

Introduction to touch techniques

When to use massage and other touch techniques

Massage and other touch techniques help many dogs during recovery. However, they are not an essential part of every home care programme, and are best avoided for dogs that are nervous of close handling. You're also unlikely to need the techniques in this chapter if your dog can still walk.

Ask your physiotherapist for advice tailored to your own dog. Each dog has different needs. Use the instructions in this chapter as a guide and for reference.

Use home massage and other touch techniques only if your dog is happy with them.

BOX 1: A GENERAL GUIDE TO WHEN TO USE TOUCH TECHNIQUES AT HOME

GRADE	HOW THE DOG LOOKS	EFFLEURAGE ('STROKING MASSAGE')	RANGE OF MOVEMENT	SENSORY TOUCH WORK	PINCH WITHDRAWAL EXERCISE
1	Can walk normally	–	–	–	✗
2	Wobbly when walking	–	–	–	✗
3	Cannot walk, but can move their legs	✓	✓	✓	✗
4	Cannot walk or move their legs	✓✓	✓✓	✓✓	✓
5	Paralysed and no deep pain sensation	✓✓	✓✓	✓✓	✓✓

– Not routinely used unless recommended by the physiotherapist   ✗ Avoid this   ✓ May be useful   ✓✓ Often useful

> **CAUTION!** Avoid home massage during the first week of an IVDD incident unless advised otherwise by your vet. Dogs easily deteriorate at this early stage, so special care is needed.

Figure 2: A dog lying on a floor bed ready for massage

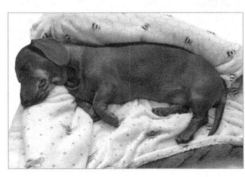

 TAKE CARE: If you work with your dog on a sofa or other raised surface, fit them with a chest harness and take special care to avoid falls.

What to include in a hands-on routine?

There's no rush to learn every technique. Start simply with stroking massage. Add in more techniques over the next few days to weeks as you and your dog feel ready (see box 2). Once you know several techniques, combine them during each massage session.

A hands-on routine could take up to 10 minutes on each side of the dog's body. Do much less if your dog is restless and won't lie still for long, or more if they enjoy it and you have time to spare.

Positioning your dog

Have your dog rest on a folded blanket, piece of vet fleece or flat dog bed (figure 2).

✓ Most techniques are best done with your dog **lying relaxed on their side.** Repeat the procedure later in the day when they are resting on their other side. Don't turn your IVDD dog over by rolling them with legs over belly. This could twist their spine.

✓ Work with your dog **on the floor** if possible. For your own comfort, floor cushions or a low stool may be useful.

✓ Put a **rolled towel or blanket behind their spine** for extra support. Or let your dog rest their back against your outstretched leg (figures 4 & 5).

Keeping your dog relaxed during home therapy

Help your dog feel comfortable by positioning them carefully and by making your movements slow and gentle.

A friend could distract your dog from in front by stroking or scratching their head. However, never hold a struggling dog down for massage or other touch work. This would make them anxious. Watch your dog throughout for subtle signs of anxiety such as lip-licking or yawning (Chapter 37). If they are anxious, pause and let them relax before trying again more gently and slowly. Some dogs find it too overwhelming to have things done to them. This may be because they feel anxious or painful, or simply because they have never liked such close contact.

If any technique continues to make your dog restless or anxious, stop and let your vet or physiotherapist know.

SAFETY ADVICE

Areas to avoid touching

Don't touch directly over:

• painful areas
• unhealed surgical wound
• infected skin

CHAPTER 65
Home massage

Massage can improve circulation, stimulate weak muscles and relax tight ones. Perhaps most importantly, it should be a pleasant experience for the dog.

Not every dog enjoys home massage. If your dog dislikes it then it is best avoided. Discuss this with your physiotherapist.

Stroking massage (effleurage)

Stroking massage improves relaxation and circulation. Use long, slow, soothing strokes with no more pressure than you would usually use to stroke your dog. There are many variations on this basic technique. If your physiotherapist asks you to use a method that is not outlined here, ask them to demonstrate on your own dog.

→ See Chapter 64 for advice on how best to position your dog and keep them comfortable.

How to do effleurage
Stroke gently in the direction of the fur. Keep your hands flat or slightly cupped, and avoid digging your fingertips into the skin. Stroke mainly over the soft parts of your dog. Glide more gently over any bony protrusions or go around them. To massage a leg, mould your hand softly around it and stroke gently in the direction of the fur.

Where to massage
Start by stroking your dog wherever they have always loved to be fussed or stroked, for example around the base of their ears. This has a settling effect.

 TIP: If your dog fidgets during a massage, try returning now and again to a favourite spot where they have always loved fuss.

Avoid any 'no-go' areas. For example, many dogs hate having their paws touched.

BOX 3: SUGGESTED DIRECTION
OF MASSAGE STROKES.

Make slow, repeated strokes over each area before moving on to the next one:

a. over muscles at the side of their shoulder area

b. extend strokes along the side of your dog's ribs and body

c. from the shoulder and over the front leg

d. over the body again

e. from the body and over the hind leg.

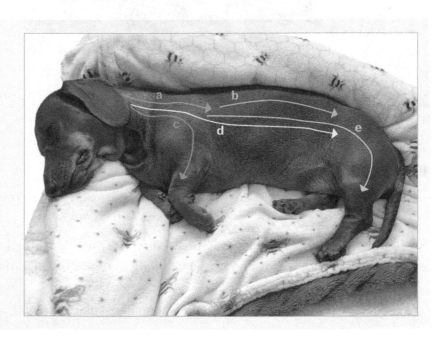

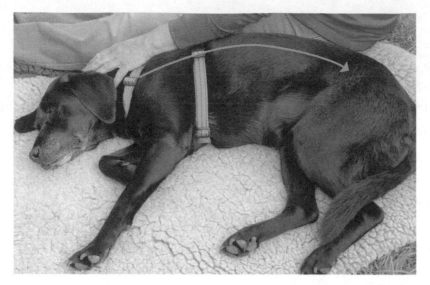

One-handed effleurage

Use this technique when you only have one hand free. You can use the other hand to prop yourself up or to keep the dog's body steady.

Figure 4: One-handed effleurage. Make a long, slow, rhythmic stroke with one hand in the direction of the fur. Lift your hand off, and repeat.

Two-handed effleurage

Only try this if you have both hands free. You must be sitting comfortably without needing to use a hand to balance yourself.

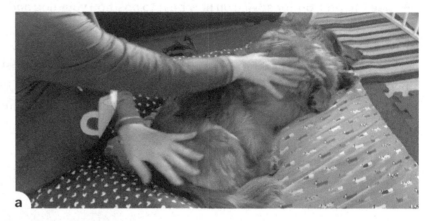

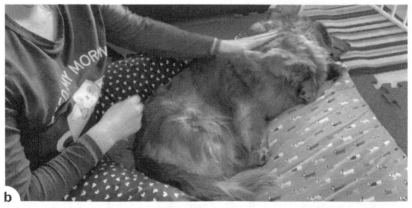

Figure 5a and b: Two-handed effleurage. Make a long, slow soothing stroke with the first hand. As that hand gently comes off, start a stroke with your second hand. Alternate your hands, keeping the strokes slow and rhythmic.

Kneading massage (petrissage)

Petrissage is a slow, rhythmical kneading technique using firmer pressure. Different techniques are used depending on the size of the dog and the part of the body.

Kneading techniques are generally best reserved for use by trained therapists. If your physiotherapist wants you to include kneading massage, ask them to teach you a suitable technique on your own dog.

⚠ **TAKE CARE:** Your dog is probably much smaller than you, and they may have tender areas.

Massage in supported postures

If your dog loves to be fussed but won't lie down for massage, consider massaging them briefly while they are either sitting or lying on their front.

Take special care to help your dog stay in position:

Only try sitting or sphinx massage once your dog is good at staying in these positions. See Chapter 59, 'Further posture exercises' for advice on helping your dog hold a sitting or sphinx position.

Help them keep their balance:

✓ Use both hands at the same time, one on each side of their body.

✓ Or support the dog with one hand while massaging with the other.

✗ Avoid downward strokes over your dog's head, neck or shoulders.

Use the diagrams as a guide.

Sphinx massage

For instructions on helping your dog into the sphinx position, see Chapter 59, Exercise 7 (Sit to sphinx)

1. Start with your dog lying on their front on non-slip footing: Check that their body is straight. Each hind leg should be folded in a zigzag with paws positioned pads-down. Gently adjust their position if needed.

2. Working on the floor, use your knees or outstretched legs to help prop and steady your dog's rear end. This frees up both hands to stroke both sides of the dog at the same time.

3. Make 3-10 sweeping effleurage strokes backwards and slightly upwards over your dog's sides (see Figure 8).

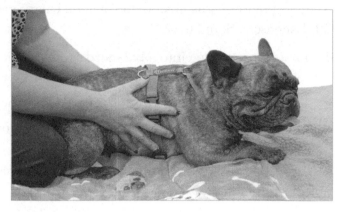

Figure 6: Massage in a sphinx position.

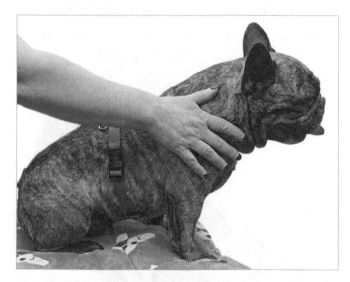

Figure 7: Massage in a sitting position.

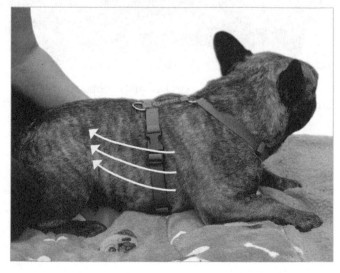

Figure 8: Sphinx massage – stroke in the direction of the arrows.

Sitting massage

Your dog must first be able to hold a good balanced sitting position for at least 20 seconds (see Chapter 59, Exercise 3: Stand to sit).

1. First help your dog into a balanced sitting position on non-slip flooring. Check that each hind leg is folded in a zigzag with paws positioned pads-down.

2. Use your knees to prop your dog if needed so they cannot roll backwards.

3. Use both hands to massage both sides of your dog (figure 9). Try some or all of the following:
   a) Use both hands to stroke 2 to 4 times up the sides of the dog's neck. At the top of each stroke, the V made by your thumb and index finger meets the V at the base of the dog's ear (figure 10).
   b) Make 3 to 7 sweeping strokes over both sides of your dog in the direction of the fur.
   c) Sweep your hands up the front of the chest and the sides of the neck 2 to 4 times, again sliding the V between your thumb and index finger towards the base of your dog's ear.

4. Keep checking that your dog is still in a good straight sitting position. Pause and use your hands to help reposition your dog if needed.

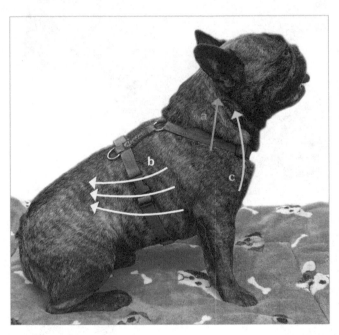

Figure 9: Sitting massage – stroke in the direction of the arrows.

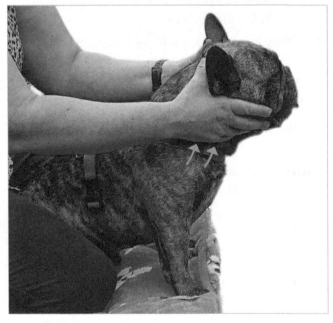

Figure 10: Stroking up the side of the neck towards the base of the ear.

⚠️ **ALWAYS REMEMBER:** Massage is only useful if it is pleasant for the dog. Stop if they don't seem to like it.

CHAPTER 66

Range of movement (ROM)

Range of movement (ROM) exercises bend and straighten the legs to get muscles and joints moving. ROM is particularly useful for paralysed limbs and can also be used to free up tight muscles.

ROM is not suitable for every dog. Check first with your vet or physiotherapist if your dog has a leg injury or joint problem, or if you are unsure. For many dogs, it is better to get their legs moving by using sling walking or postures exercises.

Setting up for ROM

1. Start with your dog lying comfortably on one side (see Chapter 64).
2. Check that you are also comfortable and have both hands free.
3. Start with some gentle massage strokes (effleurage) as described in Chapter 65. Stroke their body, then do a few strokes over a leg before starting range of movement with that leg.

How to do range of movement (ROM)

Focus on one leg at a time:

✓ Support the leg's weight
✓ Fold the whole leg gently into a bent, zigzag position
✓ Then guide it into a straight position.

Techniques for the front and hind legs are described below.

Bend and straighten a leg slowly and smoothly, never forcing it past a point that is comfortable for your dog.

Some dogs with back or neck problems have extremely tight muscles. This can make it difficult or even impossible to bend their legs. If so, try massaging the limb first. If the leg is still too stiff to bend, ask your physiotherapist for advice.

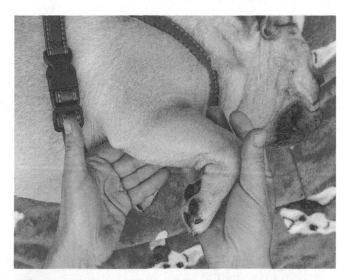

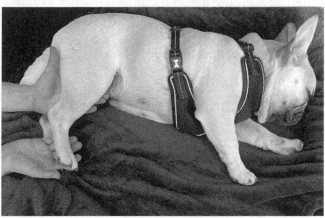

Figure 11a (top) and b (above): Keep your hands soft and open when doing ROM.

🚫 **AVOID THIS:** Don't grip a leg and pull. Instead, use your hands to support the weight of the leg and to guide it.

Hind leg range of movement

1. Support the leg's weight with one open hand under the stifle ('knee') and the other hand under the paw. Spread your fingers if needed to give good support. For a dachshund or miniature breed, you can support the leg with just one hand.

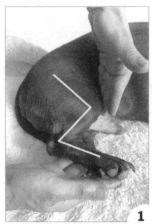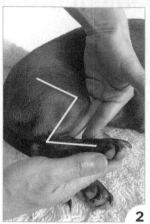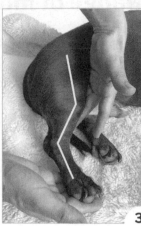

2. Use your supporting hand(s) to guide the leg slowly into a 'Z' folded position. Only fold it as far as it goes easily.

3. Use your supporting hand(s) to guide the limb into a straight position, opening up the 'Z'. As you straighten the leg, coax it back slightly from the hip. Never force the movement. Only move the leg within your dog's comfortable range.

Repeat the bending and straightening 2 to 4 times, or as advised by your physiotherapist.

Front leg range of movement

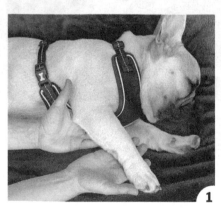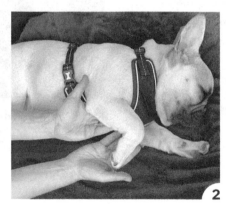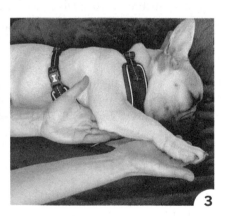

1. Support the weight of the leg with one open hand under the elbow and the other hand under the carpus ('wrist') and paw. Spread your fingers as needed to give good support. For a dachshund or miniature breed, you can support the leg with just one hand.

2. Use your supporting hand(s) to guide the leg slowly into a folded position. Only fold it as far as it goes easily.

3. Use your supporting hand(s) to guide the limb straight again. As it straightens, bring the whole leg forward. The elbow can be guided a little forward of its starting position. Never force the movement. Only move the leg within your dog's comfortable range.

Repeat the bending and straightening 2 to 4 times, or as advised by your physiotherapist.

⚠ **WATCH OUT: Never force the movement.** Only move the leg within your dog's comfortable range.

CHAPTER 67
Sensory touch work

After a severe back or neck problem, your dog's body may feel strange to them. Their sensation of touch may also have changed. The worst-affected dogs are totally unaware of someone touching their hind legs. Others find that touch feels odd. It may be a reduced sensation or feel tingly.

Sensory touch techniques help skin sensation return to normal. They improve the dog's awareness of their own body. These techniques remind the dog that their weak or paralysed limbs are part of their body rather than alien objects. They are mainly used on dogs that have lost the ability to walk.

Sensory stroking

This is like effleurage (chapter 65) but with longer strokes. The first part of each stroke will feel normal to your dog. As you reach the hindquarters, your touch may feel different to them.

Continue your strokes at the same speed and smoothness as you move from one part of their body to another. These long strokes help improve the dog's awareness of their body.

Fluffing up

Fluffing up is mainly used over weak leg muscles. This technique may be useful if your dog's legs are floppy like those of a rag doll.

⚠️ **AVOID** fluffing up over tender spots or muscles that tend to cramp up.

Make several short, light strokes against the direction of the fur. This new sensation encourages muscles under the skin to switch on.

Only fluff up briefly: just 3 to 7 strokes will 'wake up' an area of the body.

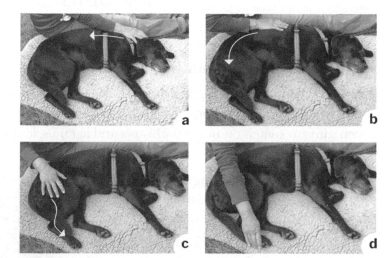

Figure 14a to d: One long sensory touch stroke extending from the neck to the hind paw.

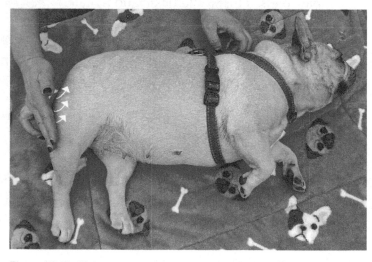

Figure 15: Fluffing up over the large muscles at the back of the thigh.

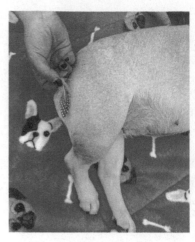

Figure 16: A feather being used for fluffing up.

Different sensations

Over time, a variety of sensations will improve your dog's awareness of their own body. Try sensory stroking and fluffing up using fabric or other soft objects instead of just using your hands. Consider using:

✓ cotton fabric

✓ fluffy, furry or velvety material

✓ a cottonwool ball

✓ a clean kitchen sponge

✓ a feather

✓ towelling

Only use items that your dog is comfortable with. Let them sniff each object before you start and avoid anything that makes them anxious.

Paw pad sensory touch

Paw pad sensory work is mainly used for dogs with paralysed hind legs. The paw pads contain special touch receptors and position sensors that are important for coordinated movement. Paw pad sensory touch aims to switch on nerve pathways and leg muscles in a coordinated way.

Instructions

1. Start with your dog lying comfortably on their side (Chapter 64). Stroke them gently to introduce your touch to them.

2. Place a flat part of your hand against the underside of their hind paw (see figures 17 and 18).

   ⚙ **TIP:** Don't dig your fingertips into their paw pads. This would tickle and irritate. Instead, keep your hand flat.

3. Gently press your flat finger pads against their paw pads and release. Do this 5 times at 1 second intervals.

4. Pause for 2 seconds.

5. Repeat once or twice.

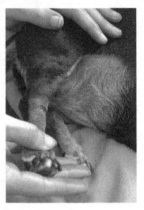
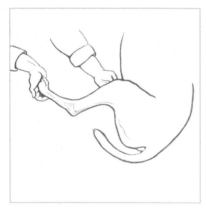

Figure 17 (left): For a dachshund or other small breed, rest several finger pads flat against their paw pads.

Figure 18 (right): For a larger breed, put the palm of one hand flat against their paw pads. Use your other hand to support the weight of their leg.

Sensory work: extras for dogs with no deep pain sensation

Sensory touch techniques are particularly important for dogs that have lost deep pain sensation. Sensory stroking, fluffing up, paw pad sensory work and different sensations are useful. After a week or two, once you have tried the above, add in more surprising types of touch. With care, you can try stroking the hind leg gently using:

✓ an ice cube. Dip the ice in a bowl of water first to avoid freezer burn.

✓ a hand-held toothbrush

✓ an electric toothbrush. Switch it on away from the dog and approach them slowly and gently with it so you don't make them anxious.

⚠ **ALWAYS BE GENTLE:** In dogs that cannot feel pain, take special care not to damage their skin.

CHAPTER 68
Pinch withdrawal exercise

This exercise is only used for dogs that cannot walk and have paralysed legs. It gets muscles to contract in response to pinching between the toes.

 CAUTION: Avoid the pinch withdrawal exercise if it upsets your dog. Some dogs hate having their paws touched. Ask your vet or physiotherapist if you are not sure.

Instructions

Getting started
Start with your dog resting on their side (see Chapter 64, 'Introduction to massage techniques'). Stroke your dog gently before trying the pinch withdrawal exercise.

Pinch withdrawal exercise
1. Pinch the skin between two toes (Figure 19). If your dog has a withdrawal reflex, they will respond to the pinch by twitching their leg or pulling it back. (Figure 20a).
2. As the leg twitches, move your hand with the leg to help it fold into a bent position (Figure 20b).
3. Use your hands to return the leg to its original straight position.

    💡 **TIP:** You may find it easier to support the weight of the leg with your other hand.

Repeat this exercise no more than three times. Stop sooner if your dog is getting restless. Each time, pinch between different toes so as not to damage the skin. If your dog does not twitch their leg or pull it back, they might not have a withdrawal reflex. Check this with your vet.

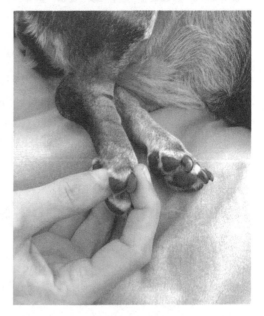
Figure 19: Pinching the skin between two toes.

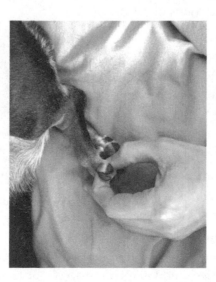 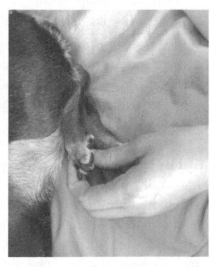
Figure 20a (right) and b (far right): This dog is bending the leg in response to the pinch.

SECTION 12
Towards a normal lifestyle

Section 12 explains how to care for your dog as crate rest comes to an end.

CHAPTER 69
Increasing your dog's activity levels

There comes a point in each dog's recovery when they can start to do more. Each dog recovers at a different rate, so there is no set time at which we can first let them run or wander free. Instead, activity levels should increase gradually based on how well they are doing.

Increase their activity gradually

Wait until your dog is ready
Check with your vet or physiotherapist before allowing your dog to do more (see box 1). They should walk well, without knuckling or dragging their paws, before being let loose either in the garden or on a walk.

Before using the techniques in this chapter
* If your dog still drags themselves about indoors, contain or confine them, put down plenty of non-slip matting, and focus on short, slow lead walks. Use a sling if needed.
* If your dog is still relying on a sling, help them learn to walk without one once they are ready. For a step-by-step process, see Chapter 62, 'Learning to walk without a sling'.
* Check with a physiotherapist if needed.

Add in just one new activity at a time
Dogs easily get enthusiastic and will usually try to do more than their body is ready for. However, doing too much at once causes muscle soreness and can lead to a flare up. To avoid this, add no more than one new challenge, exercise or activity at a time. See box 2 for a list of activities, and Chapters 61 to 63 for lead exercises.

Example: Don't increase the length of your dog's walk on the same week that you first let them out of their pen.

BOX 1: GETTING ACTIVITY ADVICE FOR YOUR DOG

After surgery: Your surgeon will advise you after an operation.

Non-surgical recovery: Take advice from the neurologist if you have one, or from your dog's usual vet.

Physiotherapist: The physiotherapist is the best person to give detailed activity advice after reassessing your dog. They will follow any general guidelines provided by the vet or surgeon.

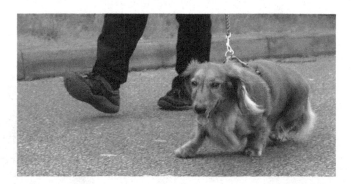

Figure 1: Your dog should walk well on the lead before they can start to do more.

Increase each activity gradually

It takes time to build up strength and improve coordination, so increase each activity gradually:

✓ Help your dog learn to walk well before letting them run.

✓ Let them out of their pen gradually instead of allowing free access to the house all at once.

✓ Increase the length and complexity of their lead walks before gradually letting them off-lead.

Jumping, repetitive ball games and stairs are best avoided altogether for dogs who have had back disease, even once they have recovered.

→ **See Chapter 72, 'A safer lifestyle after recovery'.**

BOX 2: ACTIVITIES TO ADD ONE AT A TIME WHEN YOUR DOG IS READY

Walks

• Walking without a sling
• Walking a little faster
• Using new terrain such as slopes, kerbs or bumpy ground
• Starting to trot, initially for just a count of five
• Walking for longer
• Starting to run, initially on the lead
• Going off-lead

Home

• Wandering in a small, carpeted room
• Going free in a larger area
• If needed for your home environment:
  ○ going on the lead over a ramp or low step
  ○ going off-lead over a ramp or low step
  ○ using a sofa ramp

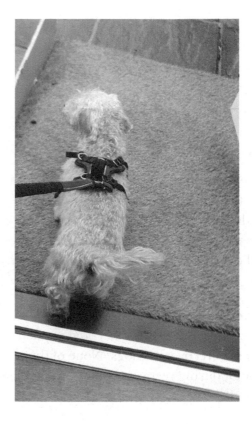

Figure 2: Build up gradually to walking over a step or ramp on the lead.

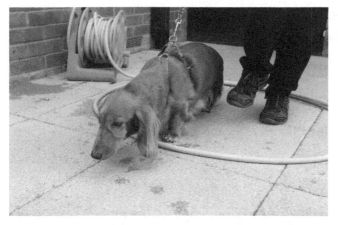

Figure 3: Exercises on the lead can help recovery. This dog is stepping carefully over a hosepipe.

Exercises during late recovery

Lead exercises

The lead exercises in Chapters 61 and 63 will improve your dog's strength and coordination, and should fit in well with the daily routine. Once your dog can walk, these may be the only exercises needed.

Your dog may tire quickly at this stage, so take care not to do too much. Add no more than one new exercise every third day.

Posture exercises

Dogs that are still slightly wobbly can benefit from continuing with 2 to 5 minutes of basic posture exercises at least twice a week. Now that your dog can stand and walk, focus on having them sit, lie and stand straight and balanced as they do their exercise routine (Chapters 57 to 59).

Ask your physiotherapist for an exercise regime tailored to your dog.

 TIP: Only continue posture exercises through late recovery if you dog enjoys them. Not every dog (or owner!) has the patience to focus on this beyond early recovery.

Extra exercises for late in recovery

Your physiotherapist might recommend further exercises. Depending on your dog's ability and personality, these could include:

- stepping forward in a straight line from a sitting or 'sphinx' position
- 'baited' movements: following food or a toy to encourage precise stepping or direction changes (figure 4)
- stepping over low obstacles

If exercises are prescribed for home use, ask your physiotherapist to teach you exactly what to do. Discuss your dog's lifestyle carefully. The therapist can consider their walks, garden access and prescribed exercises, and can check that the total daily regime will not be too tiring.

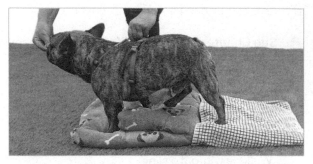

Figure 4: Stepping over folded blankets as a coordination exercise, guided by food and steadied from the harness.

Only buy equipment if your therapist has a clear reason for you to do so.

A note on exercise equipment

Certain pieces of equipment have become popular amongst owners of recovering dogs. None of these are essential and, during recovery, some can do more harm than good.

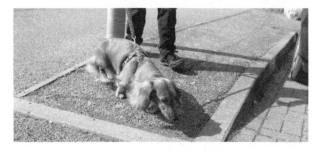

Figure 5: Used well, ground surfaces and level changes on walks can be more useful than home exercise equipment.

Wobble cushions

Designed originally for people to use, these can be alarming for some dogs, or may tip them off balance. Safer and cheaper alternatives include a folded blanket, flat cushion or foam pad.

Stepover poles

The physiotherapist might walk your dog over poles to improve their coordination. At home, practical alternatives include stepping over a hosepipe (Chapter 63) or natural obstacles (see Chapter 70). Pieces of rope, strips of foam such as pipe insulation, or plastic hula hoops also make good stepovers.

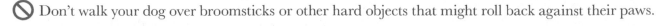 Don't walk your dog over broomsticks or other hard objects that might roll back against their paws.

Peanuts and Swiss balls

These large, inflatable pieces of equipment were originally designed for people to use for balance exercises. They wobble and roll unpredictably, so should only be used for dogs with great care and in certain situations. If your physiotherapist prescribes an exercise involving one of these, have them teach you exactly what to do, including how to keep your dog safe.

CHAPTER 70
Building up your dog's walks

To start with, your dog should not walk outdoors except for brief toilet breaks on the lead. Start to build up their lead walks gradually during the last few weeks of crate rest once they are ready for this. They should be managing longer lead walks and more varied terrain before they are ready to go off-lead outdoors in later recovery.

Early recovery — increasing your dog's lead walks

Increasing the walk length

Walks must be kept very short for at least the first few weeks. Start by limiting each outdoor trip to no more than five minutes.

⚠ **TAKE CARE:** For at least the first two weeks after taking the sling away, take special care to keep your dog's walks very short. Their legs will tire quickly at this stage.

Gradually increase the walk length once your vet is happy for you to do so. Your dog should first be able to manage the full five minutes on their feet without showing any of the signs of tiring listed in box 3.

> **BOX 3: SIGNS OF TIRING**
>
> 🐾 Footfalls becoming less neat and regular.
>
> 🐾 One or other leg starting to buckle or 'give way'
>
> 🐾 Paws placed upside down (knuckled)
>
> 🐾 Legs crossing when placed
>
> 🐾 Increased sound of claws scraping on hard ground.
>
> Your dog might slow down and stop if tired. But watch out – some dogs speed up instead. They may pull from their front legs and try to move faster once their hind legs are tired.

Add no more than five minutes per week to the length of the main daily walk. In many cases, walks must be increased much more gradually than this.

As you start to walk for longer, watch for signs of tiring (box 3). If you see one or more of these, cut the walk short, carry your dog for a while, or put them into a pushchair for a break.

Out on the pavement

Your dog must go very slowly at this stage, so you might only pass one or two houses on the street before having to turn back. Set a timer and see how far you get. It won't yet feel anything like a 'normal' walk, especially if your dog has short legs.

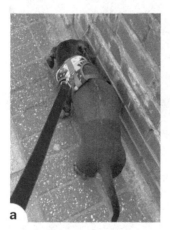
a

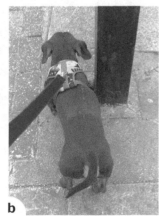
b

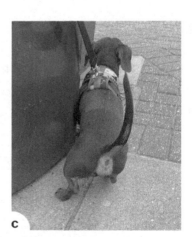
c

Figure 6a,b, and c: Walk length includes any time spent standing still such as when your dog is sniffing the ground.

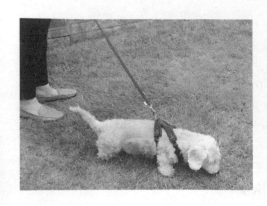

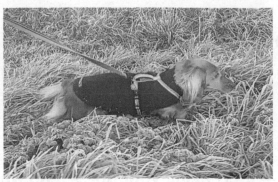

Figure 7 (far left): Short grass is a good surface for dogs that are just starting to walk.

Figure 8 (left): Once your dog can walk well on short grass, try going slowly through longer grass as an added challenge.

New ground surfaces

Early on, let your dog walk only on level ground such as a mown lawn.

Introduce new ground surfaces gradually. Bark chips, concrete, sand and leaf litter are all suitable. Use the lead as needed to slow your dog so that they step more carefully over each new surface.

Level changes

Check with your vet or surgeon first before starting to walk your dog over level changes. For small and short-legged breeds, this is usually at least three weeks into recovery. Your dog should first be able to walk well on level ground.

Kerbs

For short-legged dogs, a standard pavement kerb is a major obstacle. Start by using lowered kerbs or other tiny level changes.

To walk either up or down over any level change, your dog must step slowly, one paw at a time. Use a give-take action on the lead to slow their front end as they walk over the level change (see box 6 in Chapter 29, 'Using the lead'). That way, they will be less likely to bunny hop or skip.

Slopes

During lead walks, uphill slopes are strengthening. Stick to safe footing such as pavement or short dry grass. Start by introducing a short, very gentle uphill incline. Once your dog can manage this easily with regular footfalls, gradually add in steeper slopes.

Your dog must be motivated if they are to walk uphill with good form! Try walking them up a short slope towards one of their favourite sniffing points, or position one of their favourite people at the top of the slope.

WATCH OUT: Slow your dog over any downhill slopes. Rushing downhill feels easier to many dogs, but this puts too much weight on their front legs and leads to sore shoulder muscles.

Going over level changes | TOP TIPS

✓ Walk on the side of your dog's weakest hind leg if they are one-sided

✓ Have them wear a harness

✓ Keep their lead pointing backwards

✓ Have them walk very slowly

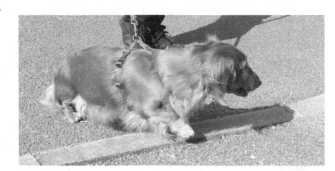

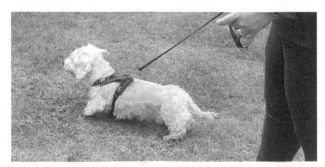

Figure 9 (top): Stepping over a low kerb.

Figure 10 (above): As you go uphill, keep the lead pointing backwards to encourage your dog to step well.

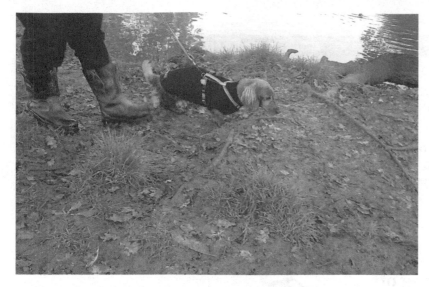

Figure 11: Step your dog over tree roots as a coordination exercise.

Natural obstacles and bumpy ground

Introduce these gradually in late recovery once your dog can step confidently with regular footfalls. Slow them from the lead to encourage them to step over any obstacle one paw at a time (Chapter 29).

Look for low, safe obstacles such as fallen twigs, low, bumpy tree roots or irregular ground. Avoid stepping your dog over anything prickly, and steer clear of larger fallen branches and slippery mud.

Introducing trotting

Many healthy dogs prefer to trot when they 'go for a walk'. During early recovery, dogs must be kept very slow on the lead. Part of getting back to a more normal lifestyle involves starting to trot again.

Once they are ready, start by letting them trot for just a few steps at a time.

→ For full instructions, see Exercise 3, 'Trotting for a count of five' in Chapter 64, 'Further lead exercises'.

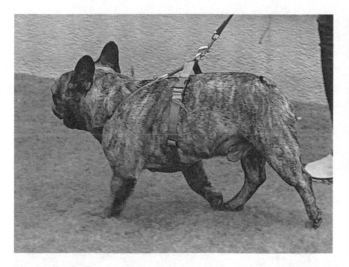
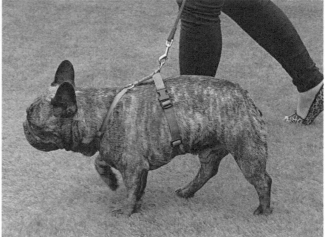

Figure 12: A dog's trot (12a) is slightly faster than their walk (12b).

⚠️ **CHECK WITH YOUR VET** before starting to let your dog trot. They should first be able to walk well.

BOX 5: YOUR DOG'S GAITS

GAIT	DESCRIPTION	SEQUENCE OF FOOTFALLS
Walk	Slowest gait.	Paws touch down one at a time: left hind, left front, right hind, right front.
Trot	Bouncy and regular. Faster than a walk.	Diagonal pairs touch down: right front with left hind paw, then left front with right hind paw.
Pace	To tell this apart from a trot or a fast walk, you may need to video your dog, play it back in slow motion, and check the sequence of footfalls.	Right front and hind paws touch down together. Then left front and hind paws touch down together.
Bunny-hop	Lolloping like a rabbit.	Both hind paws push off together.
Run	An asymmetric, faster movement.	Varies between dogs and in different situations.

Late recovery: letting your dog off the lead

When to start letting your dog loose outdoors

Each dog has an initial prescribed rest period during which they shouldn't run, typically four to eight weeks.

Dogs should walk and trot well before being let loose outdoors. For many dogs that are learning to walk, going off-lead is best left for a few months until they are stronger and more coordinated.

How to let your dog off the lead

In the days before letting your dog off-lead, let them try running for a few seconds at a time on the lead outdoors (see Figure 14).

In the garden

If your garden is enclosed and on one level, use this for your dog's first off-lead experience. Start with no more than five minutes at a time, before building this up gradually week by week.

 TIP: Keep your dog on the lead over any doorstep before letting them off in the garden.

⚠ **WATCH OUT:** Dogs act on instinct. Even if yours tends to be calm, they might dash about if a bird, squirrel or cat shows up. Don't let them off-lead until they are ready for this. Check with your vet or surgeon before letting your dog off-lead.

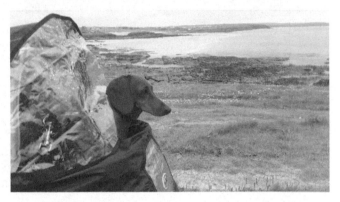

Figure 13: Throughout recovery, a pushchair is a useful way to rest your dog between short walking sessions.

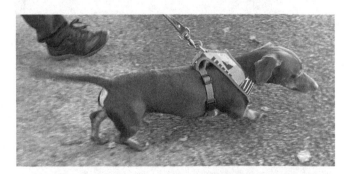

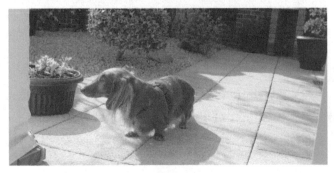

Figure 14 (top): Let them try running for a few seconds at a time on the lead outdoors.

Figure 15 (above): Let your dog off-lead in an enclosed garden once your vet has okayed this.

On a walk

To let your dog off-lead on a walk, choose somewhere quiet where you don't expect to encounter wildlife, cats or other dogs. Let them off-lead for a short part of their walk, once they have already warmed up by walking slowly.

1. Start the walk on the lead.
2. Release your dog calmly without encouraging them to run, and then put them back on the lead after a few minutes. Keep the total walk length the same as before. For example, if lead walks have so far been built up to twenty minutes, continue with a total of twenty minutes, but now including five minutes off-lead.

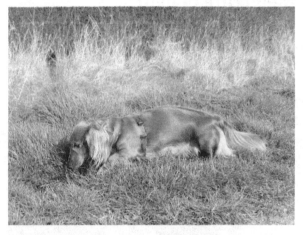

Figure 16: Limit your dog's first few off-lead attempts to no more than a few minutes each.

BOX 3: SIGNS OF TIRING

Watch out for flare-ups

Most dogs do well with a gradual increase in activity levels. However, recovery can be unpredictable because it is a natural process.

Having let your dog go off-lead, see how they are later that day and the following morning. If they seem stiffer than usual, keep them confined and on the lead.

Muscle tiredness usually resolves with a few days of rest, followed by a more gradual increase in exercise. Ask your vet's advice at the start if needed.

→ **For more information, see Chapter 75, 'Is my dog having a relapse?'**

🚫 **AVOID THIS:** As your dog starts to go off-lead, don't try to make them run about by chasing them or throwing balls. A safe, gradual increase in their exercise is best.

How often should they go off-lead?

A few minutes off-lead once daily works well for most dogs to start with.

However, if your dog tends to dash about, let them loose only once every two to three days during the first fortnight. This will allow their muscles to get stronger over time.

Increasing their off-lead time

Build up your dog's off-lead time gradually over weeks to months. If they're doing very well, add an extra minute to their off-lead time every other day. While doing so, keep their total walk length the same.

The diagram below shows one example of how to do this.

Starting to go off-lead	on lead 9 minutes	off lead 3 mins	on lead 8 mins	TOTAL 20 MINS

Two weeks later	on lead 5 minutes	off lead 10 mins	on lead 5mins	TOTAL 20 MINS

CHAPTER 71

Coming out of the crate or pen

When can my dog start to wander outside their crate or pen?

⚠ **IMPORTANT:** Check first with your vet before allowing your dog to wander outside their crate or pen.

Whether or not they have had surgery, most dogs must continue strict crate or pen rest for at least 4-8 weeks after an episode of back or neck trouble. Wait until your dog is ready before giving them more freedom. When to start allowing your dog to wander outside their crate or pen depends on many factors including:

🐾 the type of injury or surgery.

🐾 how quickly your dog is recovering. They should first be able to walk well so that they do not slip and injure themselves, scuff their paws, or learn to drag themselves around.

🐾 the layout of your home. For example, your dog would be safe to wander in a small, carpeted room before they are ready to wander through an open plan space with laminate flooring.

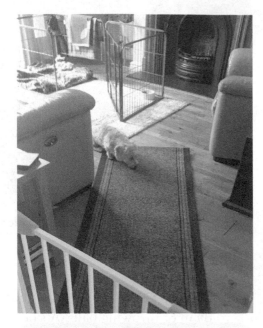

There is no standard crate rest period for IVDD.

How to end crate rest

Starting to allow your dog out of their crate or pen
Once your dog is ready (see above), start by allowing them to wander in a small, carpeted room, or on a floor covered with non-slip matting.

Start with no more than 15 minutes at a time. Build their free time up gradually over the next few weeks.

Preparing the home
Before letting your dog wander through more rooms, adapt them to make them safe. Cover slick flooring with non-slip mats, and fit stairgates if needed. Sofa ramps or pet steps are also useful.

→ See Chapter 73, 'Long term home adjustments'

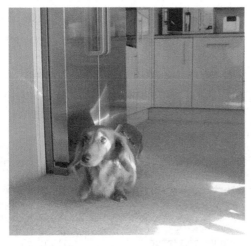

Figure 18: Wandering in a small room. Carpet tiles provide good footing.

Increasing your dog's freedom

Let your dog loose in one room at a time and build this up gradually over days or weeks. Depending on your dog's ability and your home layout, they may start to be able to follow you around downstairs, or to have free access to several rooms at once.

Areas to keep out of bounds

Some parts of the home are best avoided in the long term:

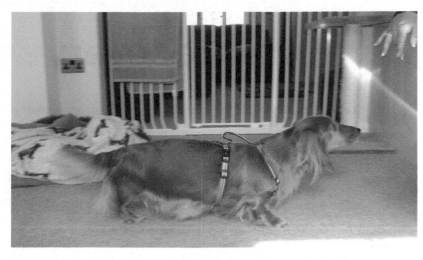

Figure 19: Following an owner around in a home with non-slip footing.

- Stairs
- Sofas/chairs if your dog will jump on to them
- Slippery flooring, particularly if your dog's gait has not returned to normal
- Hallway. Keep doors closed if your dog tends to dash through the home, for example when the doorbell rings.

When to put the crate or pen away

Crate rest is usually prescribed for at least four to eight weeks. However, after a severe bout of IVDD, it's helpful to keep the crate or pen set up for several months, even if your dog only uses it occasionally. This allows you to build up their activity levels gradually.

The best approach depends on your home layout, your dog's personality and whether they can walk normally. Even once your dog can wander loose, it may still be useful to have some way to confine them at busy times of the day, especially if they are a lively dog living in an open plan home.

 TIP: Keep hold of your crate or pen just in case it is needed for any future flare-up of the problem. A foldable one won't take up too much space.

A SPECIAL CASE: DOGS THAT HAVE MADE NO PROGRESS

If your dog does not learn to stand or walk despite good care, then your vet may eventually advise you to fit them with wheels, and to let them drag themselves about indoors. Adapt your home to make it safe before starting to let them wander around. Keep their pen as a safe place for them to rest.

→ **See Chapter 76, 'Caring for your dog as permanently paralysed'**

SECTION 13
Care after recovery

Section 13 explains how to care for your dog after recovery.

Aftercare for dogs that can walk:

Chapter 72: A safer lifestyle after recovery

Chapter 73: Long term home adjustments

Chapter 74: Long term garden adjustments

Chapter 75: Is my dog having a relapse?

Aftercare for dogs that cannot walk:

Chapter 76: Caring for your dog as permanently disabled

Chapter 77: Choosing and introducing wheels

CHAPTER 72
A safer lifestyle after recovery

Adjusting your dog's lifestyle

So your dog has recovered from a back or neck problem? Congratulations! Now is the time to adjust their long-term lifestyle to help them stay healthy.

Each dog is different. Back or neck problems leave many dogs slightly unsteady on their feet in the long term. Other dogs walk well but have reduced stamina, so they get stiff, weak or sore if they walk for too long or do too much. Some dogs make a full recovery but are prone to a future relapse (see box 1).

Discuss your dog's ongoing needs with your vet or physiotherapist.

> **BOX 1: IVDD CAN RECUR**
>
> Dogs that are prone to back or neck problems could have two or more bouts of IVDD during their lifetime. For a list of breeds at risk of IVDD, see Chapter 1, 'What is IVDD?'
>
> In breeds such as dachshunds, many discs degenerate from a young age. Any disc that has degenerated could eventually rupture or bulge and start to press on the spinal cord.

Dogs that are left slightly unsteady on their feet

These dogs will do better with an adjusted, moderate lifestyle (see box 2). This will help prevent aches and pains caused by uneven loading of their muscles and joints, and will reduce the risk of trips, slips and falls. Half an hour is generally a sensible upper limit for the main walk of the day after recovery. Some dogs do better with much shorter walks than this. Check with your vet.

→ **For a suggested daily routine, see Appendix 1, Routine 6 'Walkers aftercare'.**

> **BOX 2: AFTER RECOVERY – LIFESTYLE ADVICE**
>
> **Walks:**
>
> ✓ Watch out for tiring, and don't overwalk them.
>
> ✓ Always warm up and cool down: have your dog on the lead for at least the first and last three minutes of each walk.
>
> **Best avoided:**
>
> ✗ Jumping
>
> ✗ Stairs
>
> ✗ Ball or frisbee games
>
> ✗ Moving over slippery flooring

Dogs that have made a full recovery

Dogs that have made a full recovery could return to full activity. However, it's sensible to avoid jumping, stairs and repetitive ball games after a bout of IVDD to reduce the risk of relapse (see box 2).

Enjoying a moderate lifestyle

Warm up and cool down period

Just as you would warm up and cool down before and after exercise, it's sensible to help our dogs do the same.

Walk duration

Shorter more frequent walks are safer than one long one. Consider using a pushchair if including your dog on longer family outings. Get your dog out of the pushchair for no more than 30 minutes at a time.

Going off-lead

Wait for your vet to assess your dog as safe to go off-lead before trying this.

→ **See Chapter 70 for advice on increasing your dog's walks and letting them off-lead.**

Balls, and enjoying life without them

Ball and frisbee games are best avoided after IVDD recovery. They cause dogs to chase instinctively, leap and land without thinking twice. This puts high forces through the spine and joints.

Some ball-obsessed dogs are desperate to chase and may find it difficult to stop playing once they've started. They may look happy but are often in a state of nervous excitement instead.

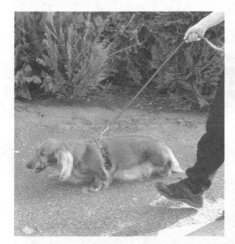
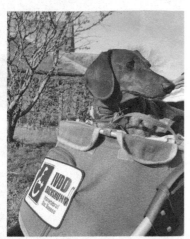
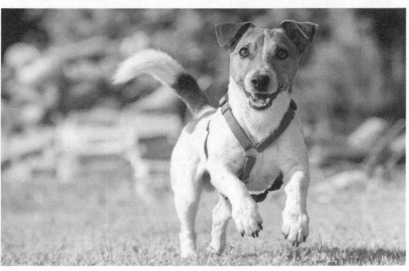

Figure 1 (top left): Keep your dog on harness and lead for at least the first and last three minutes of each walk.

Figure 2 (top right): A pushchair can be useful for ongoing care.

Figure 3 (above): Introduce off-lead activity gradually.

My dog only 'switches on' when they see a ball. How are we going to cope?

Dogs see the world differently to us. For example, they enjoy picking up scent messages outdoors from other dogs just as we might check social media or read the news. Rest assured that your dog will get real value from simple pleasures:

✓ spending time with you

✓ visiting their old territory or exploring somewhere new

✓ sniffing about to pick up scent messages from other dogs — 'reading their pee-mails'!

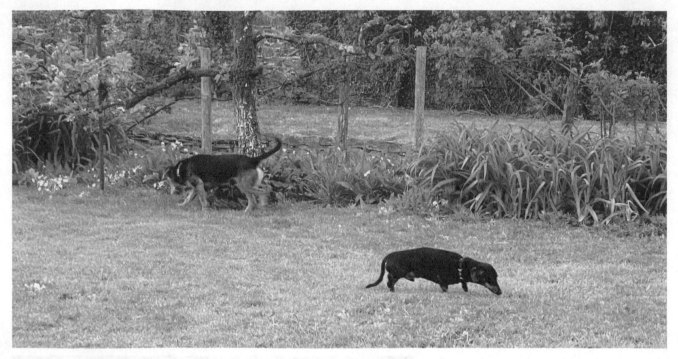

Figure 4: Dogs can enjoy themselves without looking excited. True enjoyment comes simply from sniffing about or by playing games that involves searching, exploring, or retrieving.

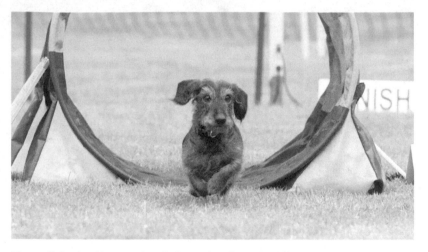

Figure 5: Canine Hoopers involves moving through wide, straight tunnels, around barrels and through hoops. No jumping is involved.

Safer sports

If you and your dog would like to take part in something competitive after recovery, consider the low impact sport, Canine Hoopers. As Anna Richardson, Advanced Canine Hoopers UK (CHUK) instructor writes, "Competing is not about being the fastest. It's about consistency, handling and achieving clear rounds and skill bonuses. Older or disabled dogs can successfully progress through the levels."

Breeding

IVDD is inherited. Breeding from an affected dog would produce puppies with an increased risk of suffering from IVDD.

⚠ **IMPORTANT:** Don't breed from your dog if they have ever had an IVDD-related condition.

→ **See Appendix 8 for information on IVDD breeding schemes.**

CHAPTER 73
Long term home adjustments

Home adjustments	SUMMARY

The following changes may be needed in the home to make your dog's life easier and safer:

- ☙ Cover slippery flooring with non-slip matting and runners.
- ☙ Fit stairgates.
- ☙ Provide floor beds.
- ☙ Provide stepped or sloped access if your dog uses the sofa or other furniture.
- ☙ Close doors to stop your dog racing through the home.

How to avoid slippery flooring

Cover slick flooring with non-slip mats. Most wooden, tiled or vinyl floors are too slick for dogs to walk on easily. Shiny tiles and laminate flooring are particularly slippery. Cover these as much as you can with rubber-backed mats, rugs or children's playmat tiles. Runners are useful placed along your dog's main routes through the home. Other key places for mats are:

- ✓ next to your dog's floor bed(s)
- ✓ by the front and back doors
- ✓ next to any change of floor level within the home
- ✓ where your dog eats and drinks

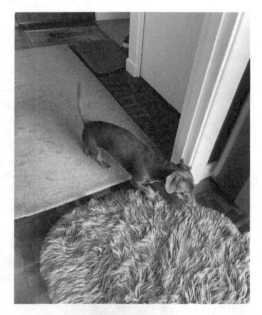

How to avoid stairs

Stairgates
Stairs are best avoided. Fit stairgates and carry your dog up and down as needed, closing the gates behind you.

Dogs that are too large to lift
Fit a stairgate and keep your larger dog downstairs. Dogs can learn to love their new downstairs domain, even if they previously slept upstairs with the family (see box 4 overleaf).

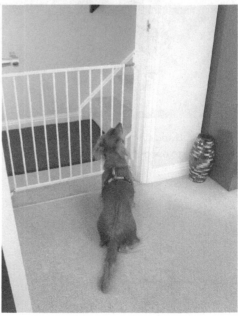

Figure 6 (top): Put down rugs and mats.

Figure 7 (right): This gate prevents access to both stairs and hallway.

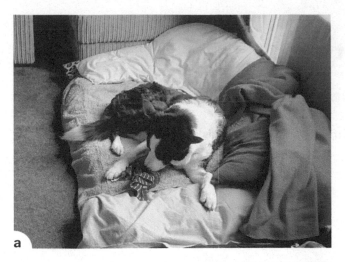

a

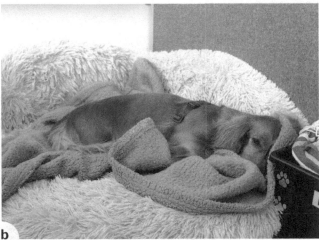

b

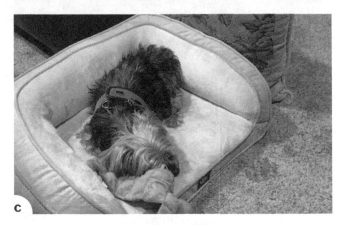

c

Figure 8a, b and c: Provide large, draught-free, comfortable floor beds to encourage your dog to stay at floor level.

How to avoid jumping

The best way to prevent jumping is to train your dog to stay at floor level (see box 5).

However, for many dogs, sofa jumping is a confirmed habit that would take too long to break. In that case, provide a ramp or steps as a safer route up and down and train your dog to use them. Make sure the design is easy and comfortable to use so your dog isn't tempted to jump.

BOX 6: CHOOSING A SOFA RAMP

- Its surface must offer good grip. Rubber, carpeting, fleece or artificial turf are suitable. Wood is too slippery.
- Avoid ramps that wobble.
- To ensure the ramp is easy to use:
  - ○ Look for a shallow incline, no more than 25% or 1 in 4.
  - ○ The top of the ramp should be level with the sofa seat.
  - ○ The ramp should start at floor level. Avoid a stepped base.
- Optional extras:
  - ○ A ramp with raised sides makes it less likely for the dog to jump or fall off the side.
  - ○ Platforms at the top and middle of the ramp can be helpful.

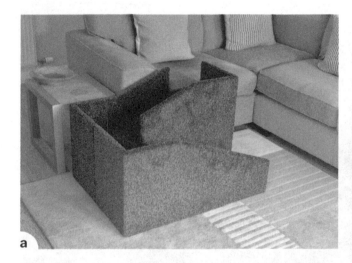

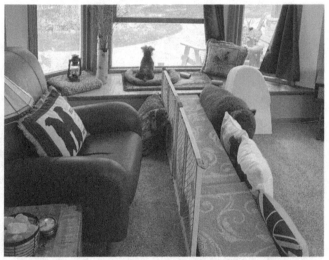

Figures 9a and b: Carpeted sofa ramps with platforms and raised sides from Archie's Workshop (Appendix 12).

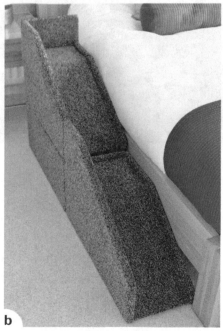

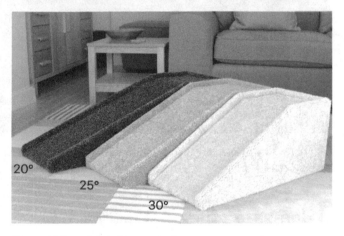

Figure 10 (top right): A long, shallow ramp created to allow access to a favourite window seat.

Figure 11 (above): Ramps of various gradients from Archie's Workshop. The shallower the ramp, the easier it will be for the dog to use.

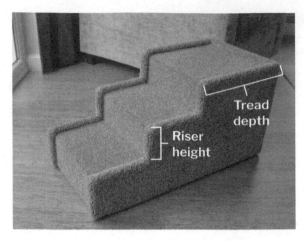

Figure 12: Shallow steps are easier to use than steep ones. They have a small riser height and a long tread depth.

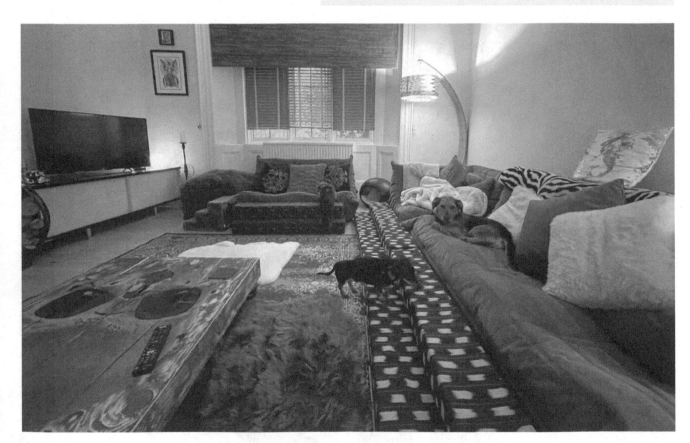

Figure 13: Sets of wide pet steps made from firm foam and covered in the owner's choice of fabric.

A dog-safe zone

Many dogs act on instinct, leaping up and dashing about when they hear the doorbell, when post arrives, or at dinner time. This causes wear and tear on the spine, joints and muscles. The problem is worse if you have a long hallway, twists and turns on the route through the home, or areas of slick floor. Consider restricting your dog to one part of the home at a time.

 TOP TIP: Close doors to prevent your dog from dashing through the home.

CHAPTER 74
Long term outdoor adjustments

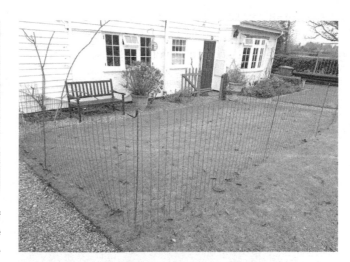

Figure 14: An area zoned off temporarily for a small dog using fence pins and chicken wire.

A safe zone outdoors

Consider zoning off a smaller section of your outdoor space if:

- the garden is long.
- your dog tends to race through it to chase wildlife.
- you need to prevent access to hazards such as sets of steps.

Gates or trellis can be used to divide up the space if needed.

Ramped outdoor access

Check the route from house to garden. For small breeds, a well-designed ramp is safer than a doorstep.

A long, purpose-made car ramp can be useful as a temporary solution. In the long term, consider having a carpenter make a ramp to measure, or try doing it yourself if you have the skills. It should be as long as possible to provide a shallow incline.

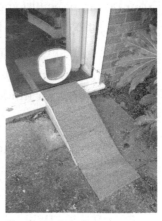

Figures 15: For good grip, the ramp's surface should be covered with weatherproof rubber (a, above) or artificial turf (b, below left).

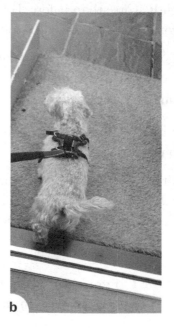

Figure 16: Dog flaps are unsuitable for many dogs after back or neck disease. If your dog can still use one, make it safer by fitting a platform and ramp.

CHAPTER 75
Is my dog having a relapse?

This applies to dogs that have had IVDD (disc extrusion). Back or neck problems due to IVDD could happen again at any stage after treatment, and there is no reliable way to prevent this.

If your dog improved or recovered, but has just taken a turn for the worse, they may need to see a vet today.

Major flare-ups

Contact your vet straight away if your dog was doing well, but is now starting to show one or more of the following signs:

* knuckling their paws (placing them upside-down).
* unable to walk without falling.
* signs of pain, such as squealing on being lifted.

This could be a flare-up of the same spinal disc or a problem starting with another disc.

While waiting to see the vet, confine your dog to the crate or pen. For toilet breaks, carry them outdoors and place them on the grass for no more than 5 minutes at a time. Keep your dog on the lead whenever outdoors, supporting them with a sling if needed.

TIP: If your dog had spinal surgery within the last few weeks, ask to leave an urgent message for the surgeon.

Less obvious flare-ups

Your dog may be just slightly worse than before. For example, they might have started to do one or more of the following:

* Scuffing their claws so you hear a scraping sound as they walk
* Standing less strongly – unable to stand for as long as before, or swaying their hindquarters as they stand.

The above signs may just indicate that your dog has overdone things lately and needs to rest.

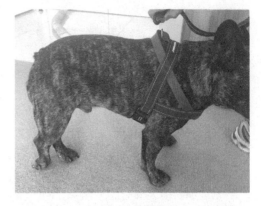

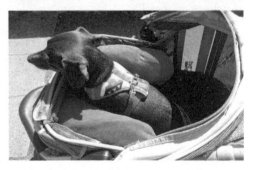

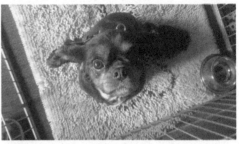

Figure 17 (top): If a recovered dog starts to put their paws upside-down, confine them and call the vet.

Figure 18 (middle): Confine your dog to a crate or pen if they are having a flare-up.

Figure 19 (above): Keep any pushchair rides brief if your dog might be having a flare-up. Prop them carefully with rolled blankets.

Confine your dog: prevent them from getting on and off furniture, going over slick floors or greeting people at the door. The safest option is to put them back in their recovery crate or pen. Cut their outdoor regime right back – have them on their feet outdoors for no more than 5 minutes at a time and keep them on a lead.

 CONTACT YOUR VET if your dog does not improve within a few hours, if they are getting worse, or if you are in any doubt. This could turn out to be a problem developing with a spinal disc.

CHAPTER 76

Caring for your dog as permanently paralysed

Deciding whether to switch routine

If your dog has made no progress, it may be time to start caring for them as a permanently paralysed dog. This would involve allowing them to drag themselves around indoors, and fitting them with wheels for their walks. From this point, instead of helping the dog to learn walk, we focus instead on keeping them safe and comfortable.

After a bout of IVDD, most dogs are best given at least a few months of good care during which we help them learn to walk (see box 9) before resorting to this change of routine. However, in some cases, your neurologist may help you come to an earlier decision, particularly if your dog has not improved after losing deep pain sensation.

→ See Chapter 15, 'When will my dog walk again?'.

TOP TIPS

Box 9: For dogs that have not yet learned to walk

If your dog is not yet progressing, but your vet says they could potentially go on and walk, try at least several weeks of the following regime before resorting to wheels:

✓ Fit your dog with a chest harness (Chapter 26) and get a fixed-length lead (Chapter 27).

✓ During each toilet break, support them with a sling using the technique described in Chapter 30.

✓ Put down non-slip matting, and don't allow your dog on slick flooring.

✓ Use your hands to support your dog in a standing position for at least one minute a day (see Chapter 58, 'Standing practice'). Ask a physiotherapist to assess your dog and show you what to do if needed.

✓ Confine your dog so they cannot drag themselves across the room (see Section 4, 'Your dog's recovery area').

Pros and cons of wheels

Some dogs do very well in wheels. However, it's not a decision to be taken lightly. If your dog relies on wheels unnecessarily, they may be less likely to learn to walk again.

Your dog will need you to help them in and out of wheels, to help them over steps, kerbs and other obstacles, and to keep an eye on them in case they fall. If your dog gets on with wheels, they can return to more normal walks include some running.

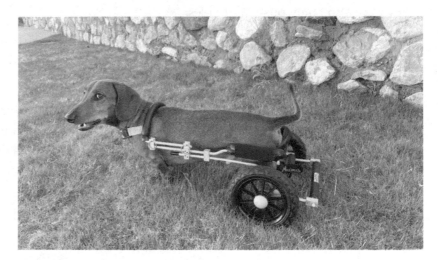

Figure 20: Some dogs do very well in wheels.

They can of course pee and poo while using wheels. However, bear in mind that moving in wheels puts extra strain on a dog's front legs, so their exercise must still be limited.

Getting started with the Wheelers Routine

Dogs that cannot walk need extra home care. Some of these dogs also have reduced bladder and bowel control and need help with this.

→ **See Appendix 1, Routine 5, 'Wheelers' for an example of a suitable daily routine.**

Before starting to let your dog wander about in the home, check for risks (see box 10) and block these off as needed. In many cases, it's best to restrict the dog to just one room at a time.

BOX 10: ONGOING CARE – HOME ADJUSTMENTS FOR DOGS THAT CANNOT WALK

🐾 Block off unsafe parts of the home with stairgates or room dividers or by closing doors:

- Don't let your dog scramble over steps or ledges.
- Prevent access to hot radiators or pipes if your dog has reduced skin sensation.

🐾 Provide flat, low level floor beds, large enough for your dog to stretch out in all directions.

🐾 Leave a large recovery pen in place. It can act as your dog's sanctuary at busy times of the day.

🐾 Check the flooring:

- Children's playmat tiles are an ideal surface as they are slightly cushioned with some grip, should not cause friction burns, and are washable.
- Carpet and non-slip mats are useful for dogs that are trying to step, but may cause friction burns if your dog drags over them too fast.
- Tiles, linoleum and laminate are a good solution for many dogs on the Wheelers routine. They won't cause friction burns and are washable. They are very slippery, so avoid them if your dog is trying to stand and step.

🐾 Adapt any garden step to create a shallow ramp suitable for your dog to use in wheels.

Introduce wheels gradually (Chapter 77). In the long term, your dog can use wheels when supervised for part of the day and can spend the rest of their time resting or dragging themselves around indoors. They may also enjoy pushchair rides.

These dogs are prone to getting sores and skin scrapes. Check their skin often (Chapter 54) and keep them clean and dry. They may need protective boots (Chapter 56), and perhaps a vest or 'drag bag' (box 11).

Posture exercises are useful. Now that your dog relies on their front legs to move about, these exercises can help maintain and improve their core strength. Start with standing practice (Chapter 58) and add further exercises one at a time once you and your dog are confident with this.

→ **See Chapters 57-59, 'Posture exercises'.**

Daily massage and range of movement can also be useful in the long term if your dog is relaxed and happy with close handling.

→ **See Section 11, Home massage and other touch techniques.**

BOX 11: USING DRAG BAGS

Drag bags are occasionally useful in helping to protect skin from damage caused by dragging. It's unnatural for a dog's hindquarters to be covered, so take special care:

✓ Check underneath the bag at least every 4 hours through the day. Clean this part of your dog as often as needed.

✓ Leave their skin uncovered where possible to allow air to reach it, and so that they can groom themselves.

✗ Don't use a drag bag if your dog is learning to walk. It will severely impede their progress.

✗ Don't use the bag in hot weather, especially in flat-faced breeds that overheat easily.

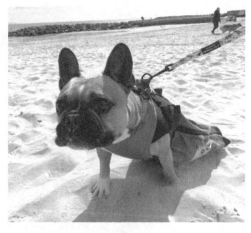

Figure 21: Enjoying a cool day at the beach in a drag bag.

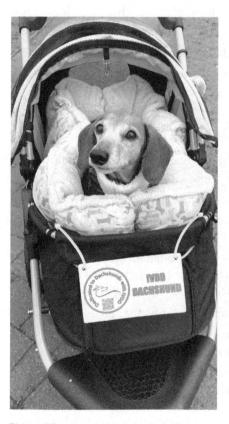

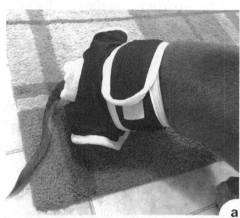

a

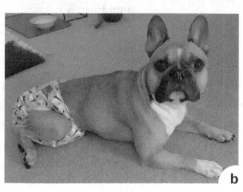

b

Figure 22 (above left): A pushchair is useful for dogs that cannot walk. It allows them to rest after a limited amount of time moving in wheels.

Figure 23a and b: Dog nappies (diapers) come with or without a tail hole.

BOX 11: CARING FOR A DOG WITH REDUCED BLADDER OR BOWEL CONTROL

- Check their skin at least twice daily for redness or other signs of damage.

- Clean and dry them by sponge-bathing or using baby wipes as often as needed.

- If you use belly bands or nappies:
  - change them as soon as they are wet or soiled.
  - consider leaving them off overnight to help avoid nappy rash.

- You may need to express your dog's bladder. Ask your vet's advice.

→ **See Section 8, 'Toileting issues' for more details.**

Choosing and introducing wheels

Choosing wheels

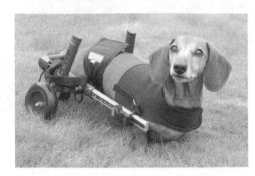

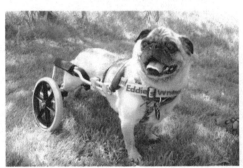

Figure 24 (top): This set of wheels comes as a home kit from Walkin' Wheels.

Figure 25 (above): Made-to-measure wheels from Eddies Wheels (Appendix 12).

Rear end wheels ('wheelchairs' or 'carts') are suitable for dogs with normal front legs and paralysed hind legs. They include a pair of rear wheels attached to a chest harness or yoke via a metal frame. The most basic designs come as a kit to be put together at home. Some home kits work well, at least for dachshunds and other breeds that are low to the ground.

However, it can be worth paying more for a better design, perhaps even ordering one made to measure. This is particularly the case for larger dogs, those with longer legs, and dogs with weak or painful front legs. Top quality wheelchairs are better balanced and less likely to tip over during use. There may also be the option to have custom adjustments made such as adding front wheels if needed.

BOX 12: WHAT TO LOOK FOR IN A SET OF WHEELS:

✓ Strong construction but lightweight. High-grade aluminium is suitable.

✓ Wheel type suitable for your dog's lifestyle:

  ○ Air-filled tyres offer a smooth ride over rough ground, but punctures are possible.

  ○ Foam wheels may be less comfortable for your dog to use over rough ground. They cannot puncture but may eventually wear through and need replacement.

✓ A good fit for your dog, but allowing for further adjustment:

  ○ With your dog in a standing position, the sidebar of their wheelchair should be parallel to the floor.

✓ Easy to clean, especially around the saddle area which supports your dog's hindquarters.

Introducing wheels

When you first get the wheels

First get your dog's confidence up. When you first get the wheels, don't put them straight onto your dog. Instead, leave the wheels lying around for them to sniff at for a couple of days. Feed your dog nearby, or allow them to nibble at treats from on or around the wheelchair.

The key to introducing wheels is to do it gradually.

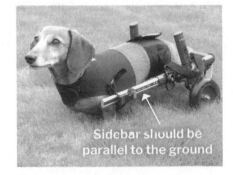

Sidebar should be parallel to the ground

Figure 26: With your dog in a standing position, its sidebar should be parallel to the floor.

Fitting wheels onto your dog

Check the manufacturer's guidelines before you first put the wheels on. An extra pair of hands is useful at least the first time that you do this, even if just to keep your dog distracted with treats. You may need to adjust the cart at this point. Check the instructions and use treats to keep your dog relaxed as you make any adjustments.

Paws up or down?

If your dog's hind legs drag on the ground, support them off the ground using the stirrups that come with the cart. This will prevent paw damage.

Dogs that can step could instead use the wheels with their paws down (without the stirrups). In that case, your dog may need to wear boots to avoid paw damage.

Increasing their wheel walks gradually

These dogs are prone to strains and sore muscles because:

- they use a different set of muscles to keep themselves balanced and moving in wheels.
- they cannot take a break by lying down or sitting when in the wheels.

Start on smooth level ground, and limit their first attempt to five minutes. If they're reluctant to walk forward, guide them with treats (figure 27), or have another dog walk in front. It's best to avoid running during the first few attempts in wheels, otherwise your dog may end up with sore front legs due to the unaccustomed exercise.

Helping your dog during wheels use

Be ready to help your dog now and again. They might crash into objects and get the wheels caught up against things, especially during the first few weeks. The wheelchair could also tip over, especially if the dog turns too fast or hurries down a bank. This can be upsetting for your dog and they will need your help to get up again. Never leave your dog unattended in wheels.

Using a lead together with a wheelchair

A lead is useful, even if just to prevent your dog from going in the road. It's best attached to a harness as this is closer to their centre of gravity than a collar. Dogs can usually wear their own harness together with wheels. The harness can fit under the yoke if the wheelchair has one (Figure 28) or otherwise on top of the wheelchair harness. Keep an eye on your dog.

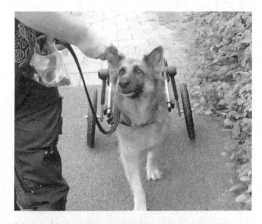

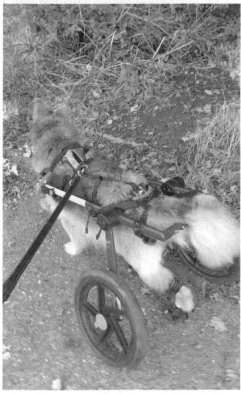

Figure 27 (top): During the first attempt, you may need to tempt your dog forward with food.

Figure 28 (above): The Help 'Em Up harness used together with wheels. This dog is also wearing special 'toe-up' boots that protect her paws and help her to step.

SECTION 14
Nutrition

CHAPTER 78
Your dog's diet

Choosing a food

Your dog will make a better recovery if they have a balanced diet. Suitable foods come in various forms, including:

- ❧ wet foods (tinned, pouch or tray)
- ❧ dry foods (kibble)
- ❧ complete raw diets (usually frozen)

Whichever you choose, check that it is labelled as a 'complete' dog food. This is a legal term meaning that the food contains enough protein, vitamins, minerals and other nutrients for your dog to stay healthy. Whether you opt for wet, dry or raw food is a matter of preference for you and your dog.

Some dogs are prescribed a special complete diet, for example if they are prone to digestive upsets or need to lose weight quickly. Ask your vet's advice on this.

This section covers feeding your dog.

Chapter 78: Your dog's diet

Chapter 79: Is my dog overweight?

Chapter 80: How much to feed

Always have fresh water available where your dog can get to it easily.

Commercial versus homemade diets

It is usually safer and better to use a commercial, complete dog food instead of preparing something at home. Though it may feel tempting to cook for your dog, it is surprisingly difficult to create a balanced, non-fattening diet using kitchen ingredients. If you plan to give your dog a home-prepared diet for more than a couple of weeks, ask a specialist to formulate it so that it contains a safe balance of nutrients.

Each dog is different

Some dogs do well on any complete food, while others get runny poo or sore skin after eating certain ingredients.

 TIP: If you know which food(s) have upset your dog in the past, check the ingredients list on any new diet or treat item before buying.

Changing the diet

Any sudden change of diet could lead to a digestive upset. This is of course best avoided while your dog cannot get outdoors easily. Once they get on well with a brand and flavour of complete dog food, stick with this if you can.

If you must change their diet, then do so very gradually:

- Start by mixing just one spoonful of the new food in with the old one.
- Increase the proportion of new food gradually over at least a week.

CHAPTER 79
Is my dog overweight?

Keep your dog trim to help them recover. They will do better if they don't have to carry too much weight around.

Checking their body shape

To find out whether your dog needs to lose or gain weight, take a close look at their body shape. At an ideal weight:

- your dog should have an obvious waist when viewed from above and from the side
- it should be easy to feel their ribs
- but their bones should not jut out.

A vet or nurse at your clinic can help you assess your dog's body shape or 'body condition' and give them a score for this (figure 1). At an ideal weight, they would score either 4 or 5 out of 9.

Weighing your dog

Weigh your dog regularly during recovery, either at the vet clinic (figure 2) or on bathroom scales. For accuracy, use the same scales each time.

Each dog is born to be a slightly different size, so don't worry if yours is lighter or heavier than the breed average. Instead, reweigh them to check whether they are losing or gaining weight.

Weigh your dog at least once a week while helping them to lose or gain weight.

💡 **TIP:** *You can weigh your dog at home if you can lift them – weigh yourself while carrying them, then subtract your own weight.*

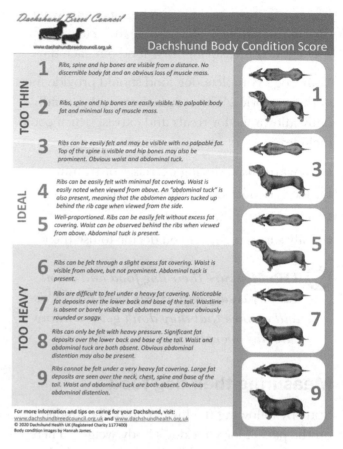

Figure 1: Dachshund body condition score chart. See Appendix 8 for a larger version..

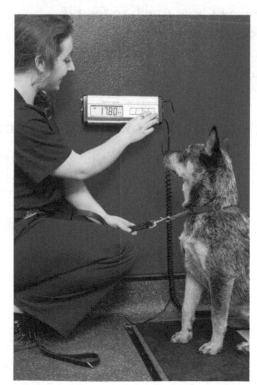

Figure 2: Ask a nurse at the clinic to help monitor your dog's weight.

How much to feed

It's easy for dogs to gain weight, especially when they cannot go for their usual walks. Help yours stay trim by measuring their food out each day.

Your dog's complete dog food should provide most of their calories. This leaves them with a small daily allowance for treats and extras, which could include:

* rewards used during exercises or training
* food used in food dispensing toys
* chews and other dog treats
* oily supplements, if you decide to use these.

 TIP: *Measure their dog food and count out any treats and extras each day. This will ensure that they don't get too many calories overall.*

Measuring their dog food

Start by following the lower end of the guideline on the packet for your dog's body weight. There is no standard amount to feed because calorie content varies between foods.

Ask your vet how much to feed if your dog is overweight. They may also recommend a different food that contains fewer calories.

> **BOX 1: MEASURE YOUR DOG'S FOOD EACH DAY**
>
> Weigh their total food allowance once daily:
>
> ✓ Set this aside ready to be used during the day.
>
> ✓ Feed a little from their bowl and divide the rest between food dispensing toys (Chapter 35).
>
> Electronic kitchen scales are the most reliable, precise way to weigh their food:
>
> 1. Put their bowl on the scales
> 2. Zero the scales
> 3. Add the correct amount of food (figure 3)

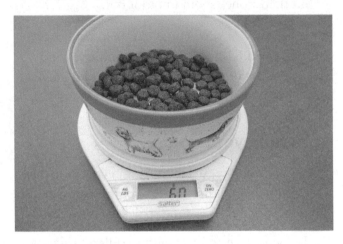

Figure 3: Measure your dog's food on electronic kitchen scales.

Your dog's treats and extras allowance

Most of your dog's daily calories should come from their complete dog food, not from treats and extras. This way, they will get good balanced nutrition each day.

Dogs soon become obese if allowed to eat as much as they like.

How to ration your dog's treats and extras:

* First check box 2 to see how many calories for treats and extras your dog is allowed per day
* Using box 3 as a guide, swap any unsuitable treats for lower calorie ones.

BOX 2: A DAILY 'TREATS AND EXTRAS' ALLOWANCE

BODY WEIGHT IN KG (IB)	EXAMPLE BREEDS	MAXIMUM 'TREATS & EXTRAS' CALORIE ALLOWANCE PER DAY (KCAL)
5-10kg (11-22lb)	Miniature Dachshund; Shih Tzu; French Bulldog	30
10-15kg (22-33lb)	Standard Dachshund; Cocker Spaniel	50
15-20kg (33-44lb)	Beagle; Border Collie	70

For dogs heavier than 20kg (44lb), use up to 70 kcal of 'treats & extras' per day.

BOX 3: CALORIES IN SOME FOOD ITEMS

FOOD ITEM	CALORIES (KCAL)
Quarter of a medium (60g/2oz) carrot	6
Quarter of an average 'small' (85g/3oz) apple	10
Ham, per wafer-thin (10g/0.35oz) supermarket slice	10
Royal Canin Educ, each	3
Lily's Kitchen Organic cheese and apple training treats, each	4
Wagg low fat treats with turkey & rice	6
Winalot shapes (Purina), each	13
Chicken breast, grilled or roast, no skin, total 10g (0.35oz)	15
Arden Grange liver paste, per 5g teaspoonful	15
Chicken thigh, grilled or roast, no skin, total 10g (0.35oz)	21
Mini Markies (Pedigree), each	21
Pedigree Dentastix Original toy/small dog treat, each	24
Peanut butter, 1 teaspoonful	31
Earls Marrolls oven baked meaty rolls, each	36
Oil (e.g. sunflower oil, olive oil, fish oil), 1 teaspoonful	40
Cheddar cheese, per 10g (0.35oz)	43
Bread, one slice from a small white or wholemeal loaf, unbuttered	54
Pedigree Dentastix Small/medium dog treat, each	58
Bonio (Purina) — original dog biscuit, each	78
Pigs ear, each	180 approx.

Notes:

- Reduce your dog's 'treats & extras' allowance if they tend to gain weight easily.
- Check with your vet if your dog is overweight. Their 'treats & extras' allowance should be no more than 10% of their total daily calorie intake at their target weight.

Using your dog's daily food allowance

Food may be a high point of your dog's day during their recovery. Divide it between meals, food dispensing toys and rewards so that your dog can make the most of their limited ration.

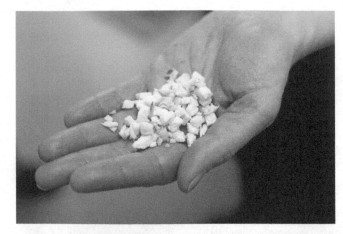

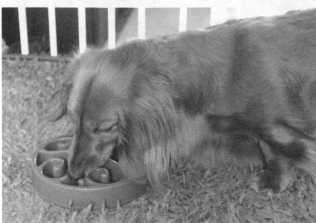

Figure 4 (top): This is 10 g (0.35 oz) chicken breast, which comes to 15 kcal. For a small dog, this total amount could be shared out between their morning and evening exercise sessions.

Figure 5 (above): A slow feeder can help to keep your dog busy during recovery.

Food rewards for exercises and training

To reward your dog during exercise sessions:

✓ choose low calorie food rewards such as chicken breast or ham

✓ break them up into tiny pieces

Filling food-dispensing toys

You have some options when filling food-dispensing toys:

✓ Use part of your dog's daily allowance of dog food (figure 5).

✓ Include a small piece of chicken or your dog's favourite treat inside for them to find.

✓ Hide bits of raw vegetable in a snuffle mat. Avoid choking hazards: cut carrot into sticks or slivers, not rounds.

✓ Feed tinned dog food, puréed vegetables or liver paste from a lick mat or Kong.

💡 **TIP:** *Check that any items fed from toys fit within your dog's daily 'treats and extras' allowance (see boxes 2 and 3).*

→ **Also see Chapter 35, 'Toys'.**

TOP TIPS

Helping your dog stick to their diet

✓ Use electronic kitchen scales to weigh your dog's food.

✓ Weigh their total food allowance once daily. Set this aside ready to be used during the day. You can then feed some from their bowl and divide the rest between food dispensing toys.

✓ Set aside a daily ration of treats and extras: swap unsuitable treats for lower calorie ones.

✓ Tell friends and family that your dog is on a prescribed diet so that they don't offer extra food.

✓ Be imaginative with how you feed the daily ration. For example, use carrot puree or tinned dog food on a lick mat.

For help, support and encouragement, ask a nurse at your vet clinic.

SECTION 15
Extra therapies

CHAPTER 81
An introduction to extra therapies

Therapists

Your dog's treatment journey starts at the vet clinic, where your usual vet can refer them for surgery if needed, and prescribe medication such as painkillers. Once this standard treatment has been prescribed, consider asking for referral for hydrotherapy, physiotherapy or acupuncture. Therapy sessions with a good clinician could leave your dog feeling and moving better.

Is therapy essential?

Good, professional therapy can be very useful. However, some owners cannot include it in their dog's care, for example if their budget is very limited, or if there is no good local therapist available.

Consider your options, and don't feel pressurised into booking treatment that you cannot afford. Many dogs recover well with no extra therapies, just with good home care, prescribed medication and/or surgery.

Choosing a therapist

Quality of care varies depending on where you go. Choose a qualified therapist who has successfully helped dogs through neurological conditions. Ask your vet's advice. They may have referred similar cases to a local clinician and seen good results. You can also search online for registered therapists.

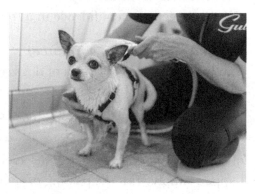

Figure 1: A good therapist uses gentle, positive handling techniques when working with dogs.

BOX 1: YOUR THERAPIST AND YOUR VET

A therapist must only give care and advice that falls within their scope of practice. They should ask you to speak to your vet if they notice a new problem or are concerned about your dog's progress.

Only a vet can legally diagnose your dog's condition and prescribe or adjust their medication.

Making an informed choice

You will come across all sorts of treatments if you browse online, follow IVDD forums or talk to other dog owners. Some of them have no scientific basis and are unlikely to work. Information in this section of the book aims to help you make an informed choice.

Useful therapies
Physiotherapy, hydrotherapy and acupuncture can be helpful with a suitable therapist. Electrotherapies are of limited value and supplements of no proven value for back or neck problems.

How can we know whether a treatment works?

Scientific studies

The best way to show that a treatment is safe and effective is to test it in good quality studies. This approach is easier for treatments such as supplements and electrotherapies. It's harder to assess hydrotherapy and exercise in this way as their effects cannot easily be compared with those of a placebo.

→ **See Appendix 10 for more information.**

Treatments with an explained effect

We can have more confidence in a treatment if there is a rational explanation for how it might work.

Hearsay (anecdotal evidence)

You may come across stories of dogs seeming to recover with a certain treatment. These reports can be confusing, especially if they only involve a few dogs.

If a dog did well during the same week as starting a new therapy, it's natural to assume that the treatment led to recovery. However, we cannot be sure. Improvement can also be prompted by all kinds of changes in a dog's care regime, such as setting up a pen or placing non-slip matting, and it can also happen simply with the passing of time.

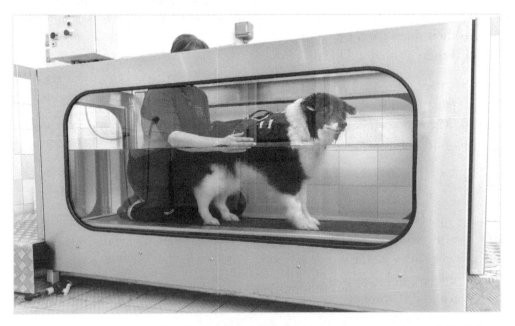

Figure 2: An underwater treadmill. With a skilled therapist, hydrotherapy can be useful both for dogs that cannot yet walk and for those that need strengthening.

CHAPTER 82
Hydrotherapy

Benefits of hydrotherapy

With the help of a hydrotherapist, paralysed dogs may start to step in a water treadmill or to kick their legs in a pool. Water has a buoyancy effect, helping the dog stay upright even if their muscles are too weak to achieve the same position on land. A skilled hydrotherapist helps dogs stand and move straight in the water, improving their strength and coordination.

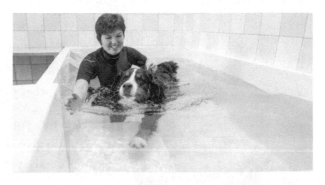

Figure 3: A good hydrotherapist supports and guides the dog in the water.

When to start

Hydrotherapy typically starts around six weeks after surgery or collapse. However, some dogs would benefit from starting much sooner than this.

Check first with your vet or surgeon. They will need to sign a referral form or provide a referral letter before the first session. Your dog's condition should first be stable, and any surgical wound must have healed over. Safety is essential, so your vet will also consider the hydrotherapy centre's working practices before deciding when to refer.

Choosing a hydrotherapist

A hydrotherapist needs specific training and experience to work safely with IVDD dogs. Quality of care varies a lot between clinics. Only arrange hydrotherapy if there is a suitable centre available (see box 2). Ask your vet if they can recommend a local clinic. Many centres are happy for clients to arrange a visit before booking, and their website may also give some idea of how they work.

BOX 2: WHAT TO LOOK FOR WHEN CHOOSING A HYDROTHERAPIST

✓ Suitable qualifications. In the UK, they should have gained at least a Level 3 Certificate in Hydrotherapy for Small Animals.

✓ Membership of an organisation that enforces good standards of practice. In the UK, this could be CHA or NARCH (see Appendix 12, 'Useful resources').

✓ Good working practices:

- Dogs should wear a waterproof harness instead of being restrained by a collar or slip lead during treatment.

- The therapist should stay in the water with the dog, and should help them keep safe and straight in the water.

- The water should look clean and clear.

- The therapist should shower the dog off before and after entering the water.

✓ A pool should have:

- underwater platforms of a suitable size for your dog.

- shallow access ramp(s).

What to expect

Beforehand

On booking, ask the therapist what to bring along. This might include:

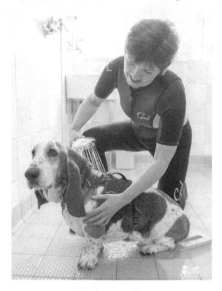

* treats or a favourite toy.
* a towel to help finish the drying-off process. One brought from home will smell familiar and 'friendly' to your dog.
* a jacket to keep your dog warm on the way home.

Don't let your dog do too much on the same day as hydrotherapy. But do give them a reasonable chance to pee and poo outdoors before arrival.

During the session

Most therapists encourage owners to stay during the session. Be prepared – you might get splashed now and again! Some dogs take a few sessions to get confident and, in some cases, the first session focuses mainly on introducing the dog to their surroundings.

Figure 4: A dog being showered before entering a pool.

These dogs tire quickly, so only a small part of each visit is spent walking in a water treadmill or swimming. During rest periods, showering and drying, the therapist continues interacting with your dog and adjusting their posture to make the whole session therapeutic.

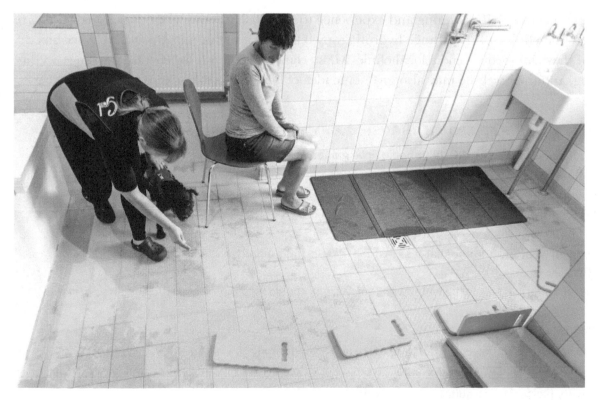

Figure 5: A good therapist will help your dog stay calm and balanced throughout the session.

Underwater treadmill

The therapist helps your dog into the water treadmill before the doors close and the machine gradually fills with water. They might ask you to stand at the front of the machine so that your dog can move towards you once the treadmill belt starts moving. The hydrotherapist will adjust your dog's position and help them step if needed. Walk sessions are no more than a few minutes long, with time for your dog to rest in between.

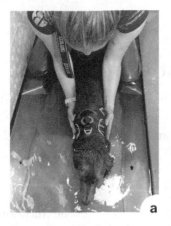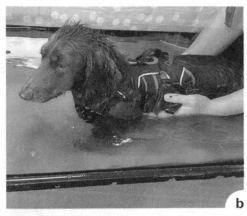

Figure 6 a and b: A dog in an underwater treadmill. The hydrotherapist is helping this dog to stand and walk straight.

Pool

The therapist guides the dog as they swim, holding their harness and helping them to balance in the water. You might be asked to position yourself by the pool so that your dog can swim towards you. Through early recovery, swimming is limited to moving just a few metres at a time between two platforms.

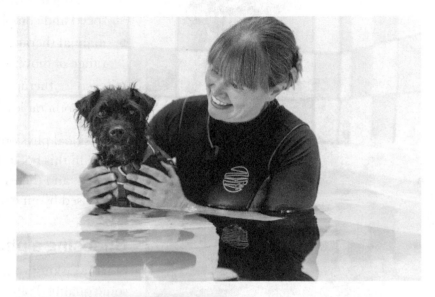

After the session

The therapist should shower your dog to remove any chlorine before drying them. Put a jacket on your dog if they are still damp, and have them spend less time on their feet than usual for the rest of the day.

After a good hydrotherapy session, some dogs feel energised while others choose to have a long nap. The next morning, your dog should stand and move at least as well as before. If they are particularly tired the next day, be sure to let your therapist know at the start of the next session.

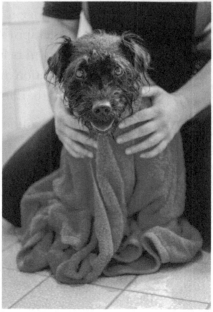

Figure 7 (above): Between swims, the dog rests on an underwater platform. This allows the therapist to assess your dog and help them achieve a straight, balanced posture.

Figure 8 (left): A dog being dried at the end of a hydrotherapy session.

CHAPTER 83
Physiotherapy

What does a physiotherapist do?

The physiotherapist assesses the dog and creates a package of care to help them feel and move better. This is in addition to standard veterinary treatment such as prescribed medication. Physiotherapy should only be started after referral from the dog's vet, and the physiotherapist must follow any guidelines provided by the vet.

Each physiotherapist has a different approach. During IVDD recovery, they may offer:

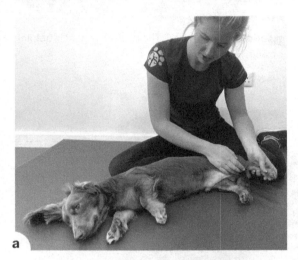

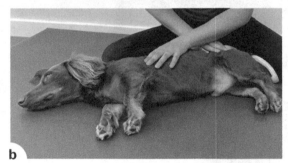

* lifestyle and home care advice such as choosing and using a sling, harness and lead
* prescribed activity guidelines including walk length, speed and complexity
* manual therapy and touch therapies including limb range of movement, massage and sensory touch work
* exercise therapy
* electrotherapies.

Professional physiotherapy complements the home care advice in this book. It's well worth having your dog assessed, and their massage, exercises and activity levels supervised by an expert.

Choosing a physiotherapist

Start by asking your vet for a recommendation. Only some qualified physiotherapists have enough experience and knowledge to treat IVDD dogs. To find out more about a therapist's approach, check their website or speak to them before booking. Skill, knowledge, good communication and a gentle approach are more important than impressive equipment.

Look for a canine physiotherapist who has:

✓ good experience working with dogs with neurological issues

✓ degree level (level 6) qualification in small animal physiotherapy

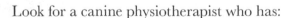

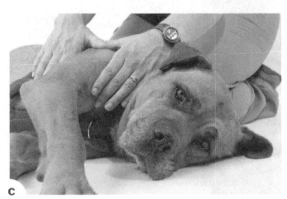

Figure 9: Physiotherapists have special training in manual therapies and touch work.

Most suitable physiotherapists belong to an organisation that enforces good standards of practice. In the UK these include ACPAT, IRVAP and RAMP (see Appendix 12, 'Useful resources'). Consider finding someone who does home visit appointments if your dog cannot travel.

When to start physiotherapy

Good, safe physiotherapy is best started soon after injury or surgery, especially for dogs that cannot walk.

For dogs that cannot walk

After spinal surgery

Dogs usually start physiotherapy in the hospital the day after their operation. This may include careful sling walking, massage, limb range of movement, sensory touch work and a gentle start with posture exercises.

When you come to collect your dog, you should be given some initial home care advice. A nurse or hospital physiotherapist might also demonstrate some home care techniques such as massage or exercises if these have been prescribed. It can be hard to take in all the information with the excitement of seeing your dog again. Consider taking notes, and ask whether you can video any techniques to refer to later.

Start outpatient physiotherapy sessions during your dog's first two weeks of coming home, if possible. The therapist can reassess your dog and help you with any techniques as needed, from sling walking to home massage.

Without an operation

Dogs that cannot walk and have not had an operation should start physiotherapy within the first week if possible. You will find instructions within this handbook for basic techniques. For a tailored, supervised physiotherapy plan, ask your vet to refer your dog to a physiotherapist at this stage.

For dogs that can walk

Physiotherapy can start within the first month of injury or surgery if the therapist is set up to do this. Your dog can only be on their feet for a few minutes at a time at this stage. Early sessions must therefore include plenty of rest, even if your dog is enthusiastic.

> **BOX 3: A SAFE START TO PHYSIOTHERAPY**
>
> Physiotherapy does not mean doing too many exercises at once. Instead, it means:
>
> **doing less, but doing it better**
>
> This involves:
>
> ✓ moving with better, safer support
>
> ✓ moving more slowly
>
> ✓ being supported in safe positions, without falling.

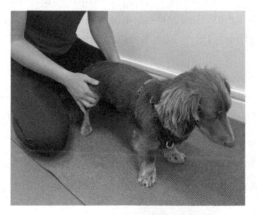

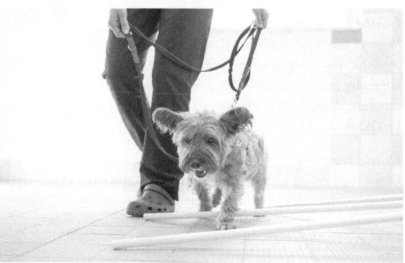

Figure 10 (left): Assisted standing may start from the first session.

Figure 11 (below): Balanced walking over low obstacles may be included in late recovery.

Electrotherapies

Physiotherapists may include one or more electrotherapies in each dog's package of care.

Pulsed electromagnetic field therapy (PEMF)

A PEMF machine generates an electromagnetic field, usually via a pad or coil placed next to the dog's spine. It has been suggested that PEMF may improve spinal recovery and reduce pain.

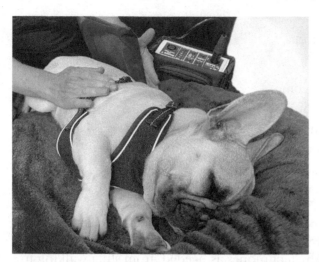

Figure 12: A PEMF pad placed against a dog's lower back.

The machine runs as the dog rests, and treatment is painless. Dogs are usually treated for around 10-20 minutes.

How it might work

An electromagnetic field pulsed at certain frequencies causes movement of sodium ions and other charged particles within the body. This might affect inflammatory processes and nerve impulses.

Any evidence?

The benefit of PEMF therapy for dogs with back or neck issues is currently uncertain. Studies comparing PEMF with a placebo machine following spinal injury have had conflicting results. Improved walking ability was recorded in one study in rats[1] but has not yet been shown in dogs[2,3]. Human studies looking at pain caused by osteoarthritis have also had conflicting results[4].

Laser

A laser machine produces a parallel beam of light of one colour. It has been suggested that light may act on cells in the body to reduce pain and improve recovery. There are many theories for how this might happen, including changes in nerve impulses and in the amount of biologically active chemicals released by cells.

Laser therapy takes just a few minutes and is painless. The laser beam can damage eyes or skin if used incorrectly, so special protective glasses must be worn, and the equipment should only be used by trained personnel.

Could laser improve spinal recovery?

Most of the light is absorbed by the dog's fur and skin. Studies have shown that the tiny amount of light reaching the spinal cord would be too low to have any healing effect[5,6]. Even using a strong (class IV) therapeutic laser machine, laser is therefore not expected to improve spinal recovery in IVDD dogs.

Light from a laser machine does not reach the spinal cord in dogs

Could laser reduce back pain?

Laser has not been shown in studies to improve back pain in dogs, and studies looking at its effect on people with back or neck pain have had mixed results[7,8]. Causes of back pain mainly lie deep beneath the skin surface and would not be reached by light. If laser eases pain, it would need to do so by acting on nerve endings near the skin surface.

1) Li et al 2019, 2) Alvarez et al 2019, 3) Zidan et al 2018, 4) Chen et al 2019, 5) Piao et al 2019, 6) Stephens et al 2011, 7) Tomazoni et al 2020, 8) Khadim-Saleh et al 2013

Neuromuscular electrical stimulation (NMES)

NMES, sometimes also called functional electrical stimulation (FES), is believed to strengthen muscles, improve blood flow, and help reduce muscle wasting in paralysed dogs. The machine passes an electrical current through a muscle to make it contract. Pads stuck to the dog's skin transmit the current from the machine via wires. Treatment usually takes from 5 to 20 minutes with the dog lying or propped in a resting position.

NMES is best reserved for dogs with paralysed legs

NMES has some drawbacks:

- It causes a tingling sensation, so settings must be adjusted carefully to keep the dog comfortable.
- Fur should be clipped to get good skin contact with the electrode pads.
- Muscles stimulated by NMES tire quickly because their fibres switch on in an unnatural order. It's impressive to see a paralysed dog's muscles contracting in response to the machine, but this unnatural muscle activity might not be as helpful as it looks.
- There is as yet no evidence that NMES strengthens muscle or improves recovery in dogs with spinal problems.

For all these reasons, NMES is best reserved for dogs with paralysed limbs. Once their legs can move a little, it's better to use exercises instead of NMES to achieve a more natural muscle contraction.

NMES is included in some inpatient and outpatient physiotherapy programmes, and your therapist might advise you to buy a machine to use at home. Follow their advice regarding which settings to use, how best to position your dog, and where to place the electrode pads.

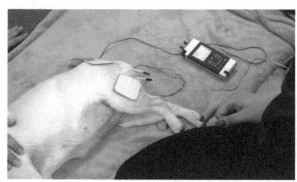

Figure 13: NMES being used on a dog.

⚠ **TAKE CARE: Dogs must be carefully supervised during NMES,** both to check that they stay comfortable, and to prevent them from chewing the wires.

Other electrical stimulation techniques

Some rehabilitation centres are trying other electrotherapies to improve recovery. Transcutaneous electrical spinal cord stimulation (TESCS) and transcranial direct current stimulation (TDSC) are used in some clinics. There is some theoretical basis for how they might work, but as yet they have not been shown to help dogs recover from spinal disease.

These techniques may cause a tingling sensation under the electrode pads. They must be supervised by an experienced clinician, with settings adjusted to keep the dog comfortable throughout.

Transcutaneous electrical spinal cord stimulation (TESCS)

A TESCS machine passes an electrical current through electrode pads that are stuck to the dog's skin, usually in the lower back region. The current causes leg muscles to contract by activating nerve pathways involving the spinal cord. It has been suggested that TESCS might improve spinal blood flow and could perhaps help restore damaged nerve pathways when used together with functional exercises.

Transcranial direct current stimulation (TDCS)

A TDSC machine passes a weak electrical current through electrode pads placed over the dog's head for around 10-30 minutes. The current passes through the brainstem and may activate certain nerve pathways. It has been suggested that TDSC might improve recovery by encouraging connections to form between nerve cells. There is also a theory that TDSC may act on certain parts of the brain to reduce the sensation of back or neck pain.

Hot packs (heat therapy) and infrared therapy

Hot packs and infrared therapy are both used in humans to treat muscle pain and stiffness. They are described together here, as infrared radiation is felt as heat.

Any evidence?

Human studies show that both heat and infrared therapy can help people with long term back pain to feel better. Warmth helps tight muscles to relax, increases circulation and provides a 'feel-good' factor during recovery. Heat therapy is occasionally useful in IVDD dogs, though must often be avoided for safety reasons.

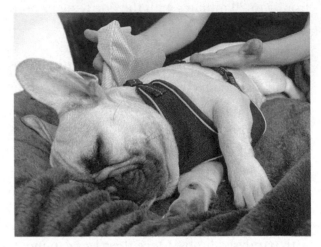

Figure 14: A heat pack being used to relax tight muscles between this dog's shoulder blades.

SAFETY ADVICE

When to avoid heat and infrared therapy

- **If your dog has abnormal skin sensation.** They will not feel it if their skin overheats, and this could result in burns. Check first with your vet.

- **During a sudden flare-up** of a back or neck problem. Heat could increase the inflammation.

- **If your dog is getting 'hot and bothered'.** Remove any heat pack or infrared treatment if your dog gets distressed or starts to pant. Bulldogs and other flat-faced breeds overheat particularly easily.

Only use heat or infrared therapy under the guidance of your vet or physiotherapist.

CHAPTER 84
Acupuncture

Originating in China, acupuncture has been used for thousands of years to help reduce pain and to manage a variety of ailments. It is often considered for dogs with IVDD alongside standard medical treatment.

Acupuncture is very safe when performed properly by a fully trained practitioner. In many countries including the UK, acupuncture can only legally be performed by a vet. Precise methods vary, with some practitioners using a traditional Chinese medicine approach and others focusing on modern western acupuncture techniques.

Does it work?

Many owners report that acupuncture has helped their IVDD dog recover. There are not yet enough good scientific studies to be sure that the treatment is working. However, on balance, studies looking at acupuncture for human spinal cord injury show promising results, with some reporting improvements in mobility, bladder function and comfort.

Heike Kopac, president of ABVA, finds that IVDD dogs have a varied response to acupuncture: "Some do very well, others don't seem to respond at all."

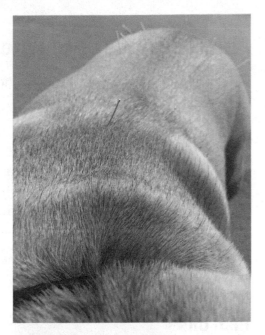
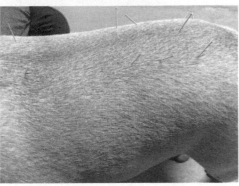

Figure 15 a and b: Acupuncture.

What to expect

The acupuncturist will spend time assessing your dog and questioning you about the problem. They should handle your dog gently and help them to get comfortable, either on a table or on a mat on the floor. You may be asked to sit close to your dog to help keep them at ease. Once your dog has settled down, fine needles are inserted into very precise locations on their body. There may be slight discomfort as the needles are placed, though many dogs remain relaxed through the whole procedure. Needles are usually left in place for at least 5 minutes, during which time the practitioner may rotate them gently or use them to transmit a very low voltage electrical current.

Dogs that have just gone down with IVDD may be treated every 2-3 days. Weekly sessions are more usual later in the recovery process. Three sessions should be enough for you to see whether your dog is benefiting from this treatment.

Finding an acupuncturist

Ask your vet if they can recommend a local vet with suitable experience and qualifications. You can also search online for a vet who is registered with:

✓ IVAS (International Veterinary Acupuncture Society)
✓ ABVA (Association of British Veterinary Acupuncturists)

CHAPTER 85
Nutritional supplements

No nutritional supplement has been shown to be helpful either in preventing or treating IVDD.

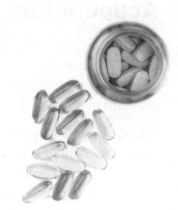

Chondroitin/glucosamine

Chondroitin and glucosamine are found in the cartilage of joints and spinal discs. There is no accepted scientific theory explaining how chondroitin and glucosamine might help recovery. Human studies suggest that chondroitin and glucosamine are unhelpful for people with spinal disease or lower back pain[1,2].

Summary: There is no evidence that chondroitin or glucosamine help treat or prevent back or neck problems.

Fish oils

Fish oils contain two types of essential fatty acids called eicosapentaenoic acid (EPA) and docosahexaenoic acid (DHA). Both are classed as omega-3 fatty acids. There is a good scientific theory explaining how they might reduce inflammation, but unfortunately no evidence that they help dogs with IVDD.

There are no good studies looking at whether fish oils help treat or prevent back or neck problems. In both humans and dogs, studies looking at the effect of fish oils on osteoarthritis (degenerative joint disease) have had mixed results. Human studies suggest that fish oils are no more useful than a placebo, and the value of fish oils for dogs with joint problems remains uncertain.

Summary: There is no evidence that fish oils help treat or prevent back or neck problems. If you decide to give your dog an EPA/DHA supplement, choose one made for dogs.

Turmeric

Turmeric has long been used in traditional human medicine. The medicinal extract of this yellow spice is sometimes called P54FP. This contains curcumin, a chemical that might reduce inflammation in people.

After a dose of turmeric, dogs absorb hardly any curcumin, and the small amount that enters their bloodstream is soon broken down by the body[3]. A placebo-controlled study found that turmeric did not help dogs with osteoarthritis[4].

Summary: Avoid turmeric. Its active ingredient is so poorly absorbed that it will not help your dog.

Vegetable oils

Over the years, various health benefits have been claimed for each of the following oils in human medicine: coconut, evening primrose, olive, flaxseed, borage, sunflower, avocado, walnut, canola. There is no evidence that any of these are helpful to dogs with back or neck disease, and no scientific basis for using them during IVDD recovery.

Summary: Avoid these as supplements. They are unhelpful and very high in calories.

1) Stuber et al 2011, 2) Phillipi et al 1999, 3) Anand et al 2007, 4) Innes et al 2004

SECTION 16
Your wellbeing

Section 16 focuses on ways to make your own life a little easier during your dog's recovery.

Chapter 86: Tips for staying positive

Chapter 87: Making your life easier

Chapter 88: Days out and travel with your IVDD dog

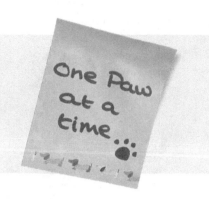

One Paw at a time...

CHAPTER 86
Tips for staying positive

Many owners feel completely overwhelmed when their dog first goes down with back or neck disease. You're not alone if this applies to you. And, for many, the stress does not end once the problem has been diagnosed. Keeping your recovering dog safe and comfortable can feel frustrating at times.

Caring for yourself will help both you and your dog. Positive emotions easily pass from us to our canine friends.

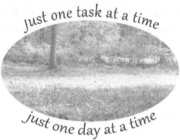

just one task at a time

just one day at a time

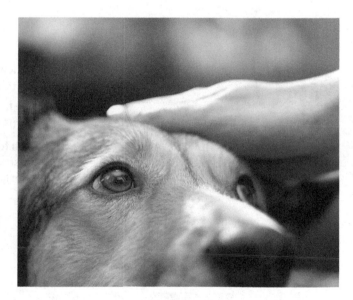

TOP TIPS

Staying positive through your dog's recovery

✓ Take it day by day, or even hour by hour if things feel overwhelming.

✓ Keep in touch with supportive people. Ask for help whenever needed.

✓ Look after yourself: rest when you can, eat well, stay hydrated and get outdoors at some point each day.

✓ Remember that each dog recovers at a different rate:

• Follow your dog's progress instead of comparing them with other dogs (see box 2 overleaf).

• Focus on the things that they can do, not what they can't.

→ Also see Chapter 87 for practical ways to make recovery feel easier.

Looking after yourself during your dog's recovery

Caring for a recovering dog can be physically demanding. All that lifting and carrying, slow walking and getting down to floor level might leave you feeling stiff and sore. While focusing on helping your dog, remember to care of yourself too.

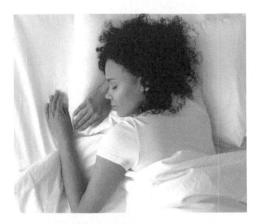

- **Get some rest.** If you are up with your dog at night, see if you can squeeze in a daytime nap, either while your dog is resting or when someone else is there to mind them.
- **Get outdoors.** Using a dog pushchair will allow you to enjoy some fresh air, to do some walking at your own speed, and to meet people outdoors again.
- **Exercise.** Consider taking a few minutes out of your day to restore yourself with gentle exercise such as yoga or Tai Chi. This can help straighten your body after all that lifting, and allow you to breathe more deeply again. As with any exercise programme, check first with your doctor if needed.

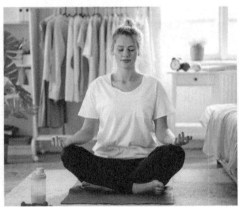

BOX 2: TRY KEEPING A VIDEO DIARY

Look back at videos of your dog and you may be surprised at how well they are progressing.

- 🐾 **Take short videos of them every few days.** This could be when they go outdoors or as they do their home exercises.
- 🐾 **Watch for tiny signs of progress** such as starting to prop themselves up, holding a standing position with a little less support, and starting to put their paws the right way up.

Figure 2 (top): Get some rest when you.

Figure 3 (above): Yoga can help reset your mind and body.

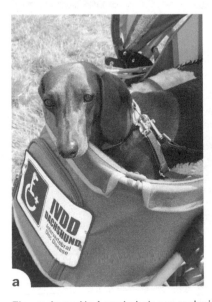

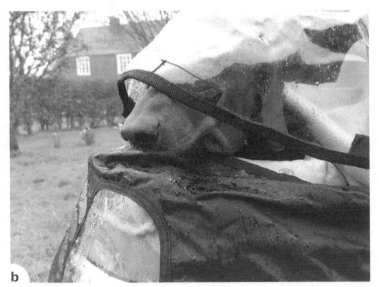

a

b

Figure 4a and b: A pushchair can make it easier to get outdoors each day.

CHAPTER 87
Making your life easier

Find a routine that works for you and your dog

Set up a routine for your dog so they know what to expect each day. This should include mealtimes in their crate or pen, toilet breaks, and all their other daily essentials.

Your dog's daily needs depend on how badly they are affected. However, your needs must also be considered. Within the routine, be sure to include a time in the day when your dog should not expect any interaction from you.

→ See Appendix 1, 'Example routines'.

Simplify your dog's routine. If you are overstretched or short of time, simplify your dog's care right down to the basics. The priorities are to keep them clean and safe, to feed them and offer fresh water regularly, and to give any prescribed medication.

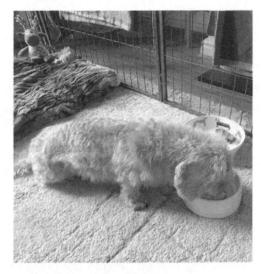

Figure 5: A good pen or crate will make your dog's routine easier.

Many dogs recover with basic good care.

Finding help and support

Support from your dog's care team
Talk to your dog's vet, neurologist, and physiotherapist if you are using one. Let them know how things are at home. If you are overwhelmed by the work involved in caring for your recovering dog, staff at the clinic may be able to make life easier for you.

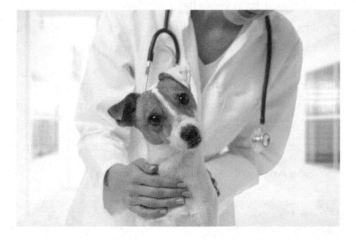

- Funds permitting, your dog may be able to stay in the hospital until their care becomes easier.
- When your dog is ready to come home, ask for home care instructions that are as basic and straightforward as possible.
- Your vet may be able to prescribe once-daily alternatives for some of the medication.
- Depending on how your local clinic is organised, a nurse may be able to help you at certain times of the week, for example with sponge-bathing or expressing your dog's bladder.

Discuss the cost of treatment right from the start if it worries you. See Appendix 6, 'Recovery on a budget', for more information.

Support from friends and family

Talk to friends and family about how you are feeling. Some may be only too happy to help.

If people offer help, accept it. Have suggestions in mind. For example they could:

- mind your dog for a time while you take a nap
- help you with shopping, childcare or running errands
- be a useful extra pair of hands by distracting your dog with treats or a toy during:
  - sponge bathing
  - your dog's exercises.

Online support

Social media support groups

There are social media groups especially for owners of dogs with back and neck problems. They offer the chance to see videos and photos of other dogs going through something similar, and to hear other peoples' stories. Most dog owners on these sites are warm and supportive.

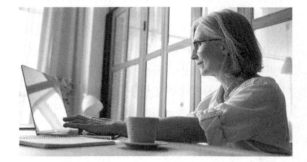

Figure 6: Join an online IVDD support group if you would like to feel part of a community during your dog's recovery.

Of course, not every online story will be relevant to your dog. Be ready to take a break from your social media feed if it starts to feel unhelpful:

- Some stories may be tragic and could be upsetting.
- Advice given by other dog owners is always well-meaning but might not be right for your own dog.
- People tend to post if their dog is doing exceptionally well. Don't worry if your dog is not improving quite as fast. Each dog recovers at their own rate.

Charity support groups

Charity support groups can be useful, providing general advice, listening to your story and letting you know where to get further help. Most support groups are run by dog owners with a passion for helping other people and dogs, and some of them have links to trained veterinary professionals.

→ See Appendix 12, 'Useful resources'.

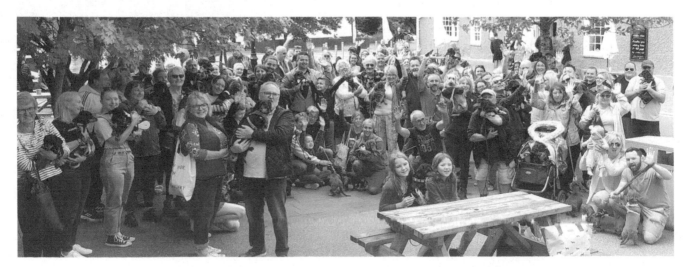

Figure 7: Owners coming together for a fundraising 'sausage dog walk' in aid of the UK charity 'Dedicated to Dachshunds with IVDD.'

CHAPTER 88
Days out and travel with your IVDD dog

Car journeys

For the first few weeks, the only journeys that you make with your dog might be to and from the hospital. Keep them secure and comfortable during the trip. Most IVDD dogs travel best in a crate with soft bedding. If your dog is very weak, you may also need to prop them with a rolled blanket on each side for extra support.

Plan breaks in any long journey so that you can offer your dog water every couple of hours, or hourly if they are panting. Carry your dog to a patch of grass for an on-lead toilet break when needed.

Holidays

Once your dog is more stable, family visits and holidays become possible.

Don't be too ambitious. If you decide to go away, plan a holiday with your dog rather than from your dog. They will most likely need to come with you wherever you go, so bring a dog pushchair.

The ideal holiday property would be on the ground floor, with non-slip flooring and step-free access to the garden. You will have extra luggage, so car travel would be easiest. Or you could consider going by train, with your dog in a pushchair. Don't fly – these dogs should not travel in cargo, and they may be very uncomfortable even if allowed in the cabin.

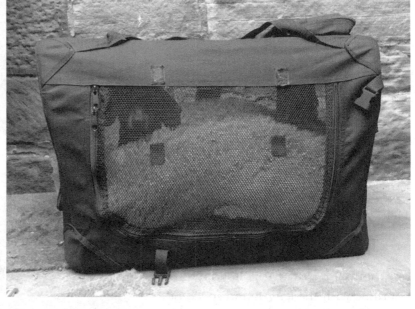

Figure 8: At two weeks after surgery, this dog travels in a crate lined with soft bedding.

⚠ **WATCH OUT: Take care that your dog does not overheat,** especially if they have a flat face like French bulldogs. Never leave them unattended in the car.

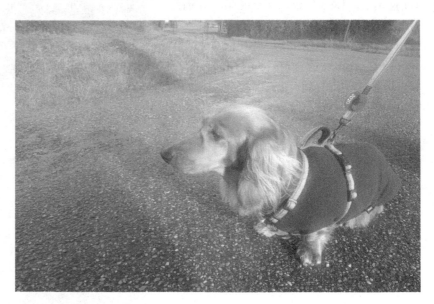

Figure 9: Continue with your dog's usual walk routine during their holiday, keeping them on the lead if needed.

Bring any items that you and your dog find essential at their stage of recovery, from a harness to food-dispensing toys. Also consider packing the following.

- Pushchair
- Travel pen – these fold flat for easy transport. Never leave your dog unattended in a travel pen as they are quite flimsy
- A few pieces of non-slip matting in case the floor is slippery.

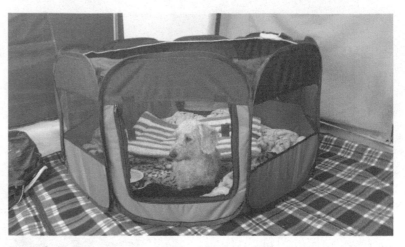

Figure 9: A pop-up travel pen used on a camping trip.

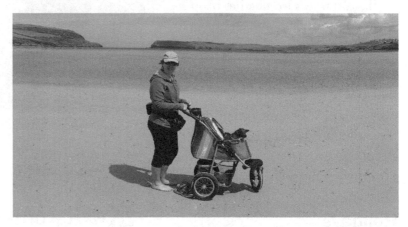

Figure 10: A pushchair is very useful for days out and holidays.

Help your dog to stick to their usual routine even during time away. Take a pen with you if they have been using one (figure 9). During the holiday, continue with the length and speed of walks that your dog has been managing at home. Time their walks and rest them in a pushchair when needed.

Beach holidays

Give your dog a gradual introduction to walking on sand. Make their first trips to the beach very short, no more than ten minutes at a time on their paws. Build this up gradually over a week. If your dog is allowed off-lead, let them sniff about quietly rather than chasing balls.

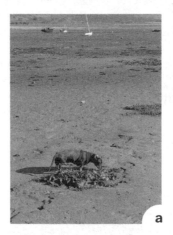

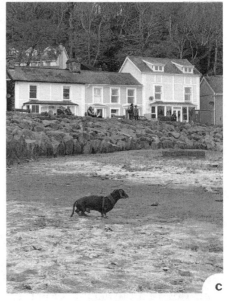

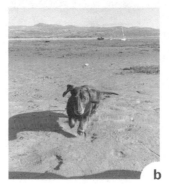

Figure 11a, b and c: Trips to the beach can be a pleasure during late recovery.

APPENDIX 1
Example Routines

Setting up a daily routine

Dogs are creatures of habit. Set up a routine during recovery so that your dog knows what to expect each day. This will help them settle down during a period which can feel strange for both of you.

Which routine to use?

Six example routines are included here. Choose one based on your dog's current situation, checking first with your vet if needed.

ROUTINE	WHAT'S INCLUDED?		WHEN TO USE?		
	Strict crate or pen rest	Bladder expression	Stage of recovery	Can dog walk?	IVDD grade
1. Movers and improvers	✓	✗	Early recovery	✓	1 or 2
2. Learner dogs	✓	✗	Early recovery	✗	3
3. Leaky learners	✓	✓	Early recovery	✗	4 or 5
4. Graduates	✗	✗	Towards the end of crate or pen rest	✓	
5. Wheelers	✗	✓	Aftercare if using wheels	✗	
6. Walkers aftercare	✗	✗	After recovery	✓	

Adapting the routine

Adapt the routine as suggested below to fit in with your dog's needs and your lifestyle.

Medication doses

Space the doses out evenly. Dosing twice daily means every twelve hours, for example at 8 am and 8 pm. Dosing three times daily means every eight hours, for example at 7 am, 3 pm and 11 pm. Check whether the medication should be given with food or on an empty stomach before deciding when to give the doses.

Outdoor time

Plan toilet breaks first thing in the morning and late at night, with the others spaced out through the day. Five on-lead toilet breaks per day are included in the example routines. Some dogs need as many as seven short toilet breaks per day, so adjust the routine as needed.

* Adjust the amount of outdoor time depending on your dog's needs (see Chapter 70).
* Pushchair rides can be added to any of the routines, usually starting from two weeks into recovery (Chapter 36).

Mealtimes in the crate or pen

Offer meals and any food-dispensing toys at set times of the day so your dog knows what to expect. Fit these in with your own routine.

Routine 1: Movers and improvers

This is a starter routine for **dogs that can walk.** It is suitable for:

- dogs with grade 1 or 2 IVDD, while they are on strict crate or pen rest.
- dogs with traumatic disc or FCE during the first few weeks of recovery, if they can walk but are unsteady on their feet.

8 am	**Out to the toilet** on the lead for up to 5 minutes. Carry from the pen, lift over the doorstep, place on short grass for a little gentle walking on the lead. Walk very slowly, keeping the lead pointing back from its clip (Chapter 29).
8:30 am	**Breakfast** in the crate or pen, and the **morning dose of medication.** Measure out your dog's daily ration of food, setting some aside to be used later in the day for rewards and to fill food dispensing toys.
10:30 am	**Out to the toilet** on the lead for up to 5 minutes*
10:45 am	**Together time** (optional) for up to 20 minutes: sit quietly with your dog on non-slip footing while keeping hold of their harness (Chapter 32). This is a chance to spend a little quality time together. If your dog has had an operation, **check their surgical wound** at this point (Chapter 33). → Return to the crate or pen where you have scattered a little of your dog's usual kibble ration over the floor.
1 pm	Offer a snuffle mat in the pen to keep your dog occupied while you eat lunch.
2 pm	**Out to the toilet** on the lead for up to 5 minutes. → Return to the crate or pen where there is a filled lick mat.
2:15 to 4 pm	**Quiet time** when your dog should not expect much interaction with you.
5:15 pm	**Evening meal.** Offer a small meal in a bowl in the crate or pen.
5:30 pm	**Out to the toilet** on the lead for up to 5 minutes. → Return to the pen where there is a snuffle mat.
7 pm	Offer a lick mat in the crate or pen while you eat your dinner.
8:30 pm	**Evening dose of medication** Together time (optional) for up to 30 minutes (see 10:45 am). → Return to the crate or pen where you have scattered a little of your dog's usual kibble ration over the floor.
9:30 pm	**Out to the toilet** on the lead for up to 5 minutes.
10 pm	**Bedtime.** Lights out: quiet time overnight in the crate or pen.

*Stick to no more than 5 minutes on their feet per outdoor trip until your vet advises you to increase this. On your vet's advice, one of the daily toilet breaks will eventually become a walk and be built up over the next 6 to 12 weeks.

When they are ready

→ See Chapter 70 for advice on increasing their outdoor time.

→ Switch to routine 4 (Graduates) at the end of the crate rest or pen rest period. Check with your vet first.

→ After recovery, use routine 6 (Walkers aftercare) if your dog is still a little unsteady on their feet.

Routine 2: Learner dogs

This is a starter routine for **dogs that cannot walk** without help. It is suitable for:

* dogs with grade 3 or 4 IVDD
* dogs with traumatic disc or FCE

If your dog also has poor bladder or bowel control and needs regular cleaning, or if you have been asked to express their bladder, use routine 3 instead.

8 am	**Out to the toilet** on the lead for up to 5 minutes. Carry from the crate or pen to the lawn. Support their rear end with a sling (Chapter 30). Carry them back indoors.
8:10 am	Measure out your dog's daily ration of food, setting some aside to be used later in the day for rewards and to fill food dispensing toys.
8:15 am	**Breakfast** in the crate or pen and the **morning dose of medication.**
10:30 am	**Out to the toilet** on the lead, with sling support, for up to 5 minutes.
10:45 am	**Exercise time.** Start with standing practice (Chapter 58) or with exercises prescribed by your physiotherapist.
11 am	Optional: massage time and range of movement (Section 11) → Return to the pen where there are a few bits of kibble within easy reach.
1 pm	Offer a snuffle mat in the crate or pen to keep your dog occupied while you eat lunch.
2 pm	**Out to the toilet** on the lead, with sling support, for up to 5 minutes → Return to the pen where there is a filled lick mat.
2:15 to 4 pm	**Quiet time** when your dog should not expect much interaction with you.
5:15 am	**Evening meal.** Offer a small meal in a bowl in the crate or pen.
5:30 pm	**Out to the toilet** on the lead with sling support, for up to 5 minutes
5:45 pm	**Exercise time** (see 10:45 am) → Return to the pen where there is a snuffle mat.
7 pm	Offer a lick mat in the pen while you eat your dinner.
8:30 pm	Give **evening dose of medication**.
8:40 pm	**Together time** (optional) for up to 20 minutes: sit quietly with your dog on non-slip footing while keeping hold of their harness (Chapter 32). This is a chance to spend a little quality time together. If your dog has had an operation, check their surgical wound at this point (Chapter 33). This is also a good time to do massage and range of movement if needed.
9:30 pm	**Out to the toilet** on the lead, with sling support, for up to 5 minutes.
10 pm	**Bedtime.** Lights out: quiet time in the crate or pen overnight.

When they are ready

→ Switch to routine 1 (Movers and improvers) once your dog can walk.

Daily routine 3: Leaky learners

This is a starter routine for dogs that cannot walk and have reduced bladder or bowel control:

- ❀ dogs with severe IVDD
- ❀ dogs with severe traumatic disc or FCE

Routine 3 includes clean-ups, bedding changes and expressing their bladder.

Notes for routine 3

✓ **Water.** If your dog cannot move about easily, bring water to them every couple of hours during the day.

✓ **Bladder expression**, if needed, is usually done three times daily.

✓ **Medication** is given three times daily in this example routine. If dosing twice daily, then instead give their medication every twelve hours, for example at 8 am and 8 pm. You may need to adjust the times of their doses slightly. For example, some types of bladder tablets are best given 30 to 60 minutes before expressing the dog's bladder.

✓ **Turn your dog** at least every four hours during the day if needed (ask your vet, and see Chapter 55).

✓ **Nappies or belly bands**, if used, should be removed whenever your dog goes outdoors. This gives them a chance to pee and poo normally and allows fresh air to reach their skin.

7:15 am	**Out to the toilet** for up to 5 minutes: Carry from the crate/pen to the lawn. Support their rear end with a sling and allow them to walk slowly. Give them the chance to try to pee and poo. If your vet has advised you to do so, **express their bladder**. Carry them back indoors. → Check them for sore or dirty areas. Sponge bathe if needed or use a baby wipe. Change bedding if needed. Then return to the crate/pen.
7:30 am	**Breakfast** in the crate or pen, and the morning dose of **medication.**
10:30 am	**Out to the toilet** on the lead, with sling support, for up to 5 minutes (see 7:15 am).
10:45 am	**Exercise time.** Start with standing practice (chapter 58) or exercises prescribed by your physiotherapist.
11 am	**Massage**, range of movement and sensory touch work (Section 11) Return to the pen where there are a few bits of kibble within easy reach.
1 pm	Offer a snuffle mat in the pen to keep your dog occupied while you eat lunch.
2:30 pm	**Out to the toilet** on the lead, with sling support, for up to 5 minutes. **Express their bladder** if needed (see 7:15 am). Wipe them clean if needed and check that their bedding is clean and dry.
3:30 pm	Give **medication** (if prescribed 3 times daily).
4 to 5 pm	**Quiet time** when your dog should not expect much interaction with you.
5:15 am	**Evening meal.** Offer a small meal in a bowl in the pen.
5:30 pm	**Out to the toilet** on the lead with sling support, for up to 5 minutes
5:45 pm	**Exercise time** (see 10:45 am) Check that your dog and their bedding are clean, then return them to the pen where there is a snuffle mat.
7 pm	Offer a lick mat in the pen while you eat your dinner
8:30 pm	**Together time** for up to 30 minutes (optional). Sit quietly with your dog while keeping hold of their harness (Chapter 32). This can be a good time for more **massage** and range of movement if needed (see 11 am) It's also a good time to **check the surgical wound** if your dog has had an operation (Chapter 33).
9:30 pm	**Out to the toilet** on the lead, with sling support, for up to 5 minutes. Check that your dog and their bedding are clean, then return them to the crate/pen.
9:45 pm	Measure out your dog's food ready for tomorrow.
11:30 pm	Night-time dose of **medication**
11:40 pm	**Express bladder** if needed. Wipe them clean and check that bedding is clean and dry.
12am	**Bedtime.** Quiet time overnight in the crate or pen.

When they are ready

→ Switch to routine 2 (Learner dogs) once your dog can pee and poo outdoors again.

→ Switch to routine 1 (Movers and improvers) when your dog becomes able to walk.

→ Switch to routine 5 (Wheelers) for ongoing care in wheels if your dog does not learn to walk again, but only after discussion with your vet. See Chapters 76 and 77.

Routine 4: Graduates – starting to let your dog out of the crate

The Graduates routine is used towards the end of the crate rest or pen rest period. Check with your vet before starting this routine. It involves a little wandering outside the crate, and slightly more outdoor activity.

8 am	**Out to the toilet** on the lead for 5 minutes: help them out of the crate or pen, walk on the lead to the back door over non-slip matting, lift over any steps, go slowly on the lead for a chance to pee and poo.
8:10 am	Measure out your dog's daily ration of food, setting some aside for dinner and for any food-dispensing toys.
8:15 am	**Breakfast** in the crate or pen. Measure out your dog's daily ration of food, setting some aside to be used later in the day for rewards and to fill food dispensing toys.
10:30 am	**Out for a walk and pushchair ride.** For example, 10 minutes walking, then 15 minutes in the pushchair, then 5 minutes walking* Return to the pen where there is a little kibble scattered over the floor.
12:30 pm	Allow to wander about, supervised, in a room with non-slip flooring for 15 minutes. A small, carpeted room is perfect. Don't allow them to jump on or off furniture or to use steps.
1:30 pm	Offer a snuffle mat in the crate or pen to keep your dog occupied while you eat lunch.
2 pm	**Out to the toilet** on the lead for 5 minutes (see 8 am) Return them to the pen where there is a filled Kong.
2:30 to 4:30 pm	**Quiet time** when your dog should not expect much interaction with you.
4:30 pm	Allow to wander, supervised, in a room with non-slip flooring for 15 minutes (see 12:30 pm). Return to the pen where there is a snuffle mat.
5:15 pm	**Evening meal** in a bowl in the crate or pen.
6 pm	**Out for a walk and pushchair ride.** For example, 5 minutes walking, then 20 minutes in the pushchair, then 5 minutes walking*
7 pm	Offer a lick mat in the crate or pen while you eat your dinner.
9:30 pm	**Out to the toilet** on the lead for 5 minutes (see 8 am).
10 pm	**Bedtime:** quiet time overnight in the crate or pen.

*Increase your dog's walks gradually (Chapter 70)

When they are ready

→ See Chapter 71 for advice on increasing your dog's freedom.
→ Once your dog no longer needs a crate or pen, switch to routine 6 (Walkers aftercare).

Routine 5: Wheelers – permanently paralysed dogs

This is an aftercare routine for dogs that still cannot walk and are now using wheels. Check first with your vet before switching to this routine (Chapter 76).

8:10 am	Measure out your dog's daily ration of food, setting some aside for dinner and for any food-dispensing toys.
8:15 am	**Breakfast**
8:30 am	**Out to the toilet:** help your dog into their wheels and let them out into the garden, helping them over the step or ramp as needed. Keep an eye on them in case their cart gets stuck or tips over. Leave their belly band or nappy off whenever outdoors. Express their bladder and help them to poo if needed.
8:45 am	Back indoors, check them for sore or dirty skin. Sponge bathe if needed or use a baby wipe. Put on a fresh belly band or nappy. Change their bedding if wet.
9 am	**Exercise time**, if recommended by your physiotherapist (see Chapters 57 to 59)
9:30 am	Free time indoors. Have your dog wear a drag bag, vest and/or protective boots if needed to protect their skin. Close doors so they don't rush to the front door.
10:30 am	**Out for a pushchair ride with you** and/or a walk in their wheels.
11:30 am	Optional: massage time and range of movement
12 pm	Free time indoors (see 9:30 am)
2 pm	**Out to the toilet** in wheels in the garden (see 8:30 am). If needed, **express their bladder** and help them to poo.
2:15 pm	Wipe them clean if needed and check skin for sores. Put on a clean belly band or nappy.
2:30 pm	Free time indoors (see 9:30 am)
5:15 pm	**Evening meal**
5:30 pm	**Out to the toilet** in wheels in the garden (see 8:30 am).
5:45 pm	Free time indoors (see 9:30 am)
8:30 pm	Optional: massage time and range of movement
9:30 pm	**Out to the toilet** in wheels in the garden (see 8:30 am). If needed, **express their bladder** and help them to poo.
10 pm	**Bedtime.** Wipe them clean if needed and check that their bedding is dry before saying goodnight. To help avoid skin infections, leave their nappy or belly band off overnight.

When they are ready

→ See Chapter 71 for advice on increasing your dog's freedom.

→ Once your dog no longer needs a crate or pen, switch to routine 6 (Walkers aftercare).

Routine 6: Walkers aftercare

This is an aftercare routine for dogs with longer term issues. They can walk without falling but are still slightly unsteady on their feet. Check with your vet before starting routine 6: it includes some off-lead time outdoors and does not use a crate or pen.

8 am	**Out to the toilet** for up to 10 minutes for a chance to pee and poo. Help them over the doorstep if needed. Keep your dog on the lead if needed (check with your vet).
8:10 am	Measure out your dog's daily ration of food, setting some aside for dinner and for any food-dispensing toys.
8:15 am	**Breakfast**. Your dog should be on non-slip footing for this.
9 am	Free time indoors within a safe part of the house. Avoid slick floors, jumping and stairs. Close doors to stop your dog rushing through the home in response to the doorbell.
10:30 am	**Out for a walk**. Keep them on the lead for at least the first and last few minutes of the walk. Walk length depends on your dog's needs but is typically no more than 30 minutes (check with your vet). Many dogs should be on their feet for no longer than 10 minutes at a time. A pushchair may be useful.
11 am	Free time indoors (see 9 am). Food-dispensing toys are useful, especially while you are eating, or if you need to go out and leave your dog.
4 pm	**Out for a walk** (see 10:30 am). Two shorter walks per day are better than one long one.
4:30 pm	Free time indoors (see 9 am)
5:30 pm	**Evening meal**. Your dog should be on non-slip footing for this.
6 pm	**Out to the toilet** (see 8 am)
6:15 pm	Free time indoors (see 9 am)
9:30 pm	**Out to the toilet** (see 8 am)
10 pm	**Bedtime**. A large flat floor bed without raised edges is best. Non-slip matting around the bed will help your dog to stay safe when they get up.

APPENDIX 2
Shopping lists

You may need the following equipment during your dog's recovery. The biggest initial outlay will probably be for the recovery crate or pen.

LIST 1: For all dogs

Essentials

✓ Pen or crate suitable for your dog's size (Chapter 17)

✓ For setting up the crate or pen:
  - Bedding: a flat low dog bed without raised edges, or a crate mat or crate pad (Chapter 22).
  - Absorbent, machine-washable top layer bedding. Blankets are suitable for all dogs. Vet fleece or fluffy bathmats are suitable for females and neutered male dogs.
  - Water bowl to fit neatly in the corner of the pen or clip to the inside of the crate.
  - Non-slip matting to cover the base of the crate or pen (not needed if placing a pen on carpet).
  - Rolled towels, rolled blankets or a cot bumper for blocking off any draughts.

✓ To keep your dog safe outside the crate or pen:
  - A fixed-length dog lead (Chapter 27)
  - A chest harness that fits your dog, preferably with a Y-shaped front (Chapter 26)
  - Hindquarter sling if your dog cannot walk (Chapter 28)
  - Non-slip matting for the home if your floors are slick (rugs, mats and/or runners)

Recommended extras

✓ Food-dispensing toys: the lick mat and snuffle mat are safest for the first few weeks.

✓ A dog pushchair (stroller) (Chapter 36)

LIST 2: Extras for incontinent dogs

✓ Extra pieces of washable bedding (vet fleece, bathmats or blankets) to make washing easier.

✓ Incontinence pads ('pee pads')

✓ Plastic sheeting such as large bin liners to protect your floor under the crate and to protect your dog's mattress if they are using one.

✓ Equipment for cleaning and drying your dog (Chapter 51). You may find the following useful:

  - Unscented baby wipes (for small clean-ups)
  - Spray-bottle of water
  - Cloths, sponges and a bowl for water
  - Plenty of old towels

✓ Optional: Belly bands for male dogs, nappies for female dogs (Chapter 52)

LIST 3: Extras for certain situations

✓ **After an operation**: your dog may need an Elizabethan collar (cone) and/or a pet shirt. Veterinary staff will advise you and can usually supply these.

✓ **If advised by your vet or surgeon**: specialised padding or a recovery mattress to fit the entire base of the crate or pen.

✓ **For taller dogs** once they can stand: raised food and water bowls.

✓ **For anxious dogs**: Adaptil diffuser (Chapter 34).

✓ **If paws are damaged**: protective boots may be needed (Chapter 56)

APPENDIX 3
Clinical grade charts

Dogs with a disc extrusion (Hansen type 1 IVDD) affecting their back are graded out of 5 based on their clinical signs. Grade 5 dogs have the most severe signs and are less likely to recover.

CLINICAL GRADE CHART FOR DOGS WITH A DISC EXTRUSION AFFECTING THEIR BACK

CLINICAL GRADE	HOW DOES THE DOG LOOK?			
1	painful			
2	painful	wobbly walking		
3	painful	cannot walk		
4	painful	cannot walk	paralysed legs	Reduced bladder and bowel control
5	painful	cannot walk	paralysed legs	Reduced bladder and bowel control	cannot feel their toes

Chances of recovery for dogs with a disc extrusion affecting their back

Typical chances of recovery are shown here for dogs with each grade, as based on the results of studies. Grade 1 dogs are generally said to have recovered once pain has resolved. Grade 2 to 5 dogs are considered to have recovered once they are also able to walk.

CLINICAL GRADE	APPROXIMATE CHANCE OF RECOVERY	
	WITH NON-SURGICAL CARE	AFTER SPINAL SURGERY
1	80% [2,3,8,9]	80% to 95% [1,6,11]
2	80% [2,3,8,9]	95% [1,4,5,6,10]
3	80% [7]	95% [7]
4	64% * [7,12]	90% [7]
5	10% * [7]	60% [7]

*These results were based on small numbers of cases, and it is possible that recovery rates may be higher than this. Further studies are currently looking more closely at non-surgical recovery.

1) Aikawa et al 2012, 2) Davies & Sharp 1983, 3) Hayashi et al 2007, 4) Ingram et al 2013, 5) Jeong et al 2018, 6) Kazakos et al 2005, 7) Langerhuus & Miles 2017, 8) Levine et al 2007, 9) Mann et al 2007, 10) Nečas 1999, 11) Sukhiani et al 1996, 12) Sedlacek et al 2022

Further notes

- Some dogs are left with a slightly wobbly gait or with imperfect bladder or bowel control, even if they are considered to have recovered successfully.

- Dogs that don't recover the ability to walk may in some cases go on to live a happy life in wheels.

- See Appendix 11 for a list of full references.

Myelomalacia

During the first week of severe IVDD, a few dogs get much worse due to a problem called myelomalacia. In these unlucky dogs, part of the spinal cord loses its normal blood supply and becomes softened and permanently damaged. This can happen even after what seemed to be a successful surgery.

There is a type of myelomalacia that gets worse and worse. This is called **progressive myelomalacia** or **PMM**. In dogs with PMM, damage moves up the spinal cord towards the dog's head. Affected dogs become increasingly painful and distressed, and the condition is not treatable. Unfortunately, the only kind way forward for these dogs is euthanasia.

PMM affects around one in seven dogs that have IVDD and no deep pain sensation. It is very unlikely to happen in dogs that do have deep pain sensation.

APPENDIX 4
Crate and pen sizes

Standard crate sizes

Crates are sold in standard sizes. Exact measurements vary slightly between brands.

CRATE SIZE	INCHES			CENTIMETRES		
	LENGTH	WIDTH	HEIGHT	LENGTH	WIDTH	HEIGHT
M	30	21	23.5	76	53	60
L	36	22.7	25	92.5	57.5	64
XL	42	28.5	31.5	106	70	80
XXL	48	29	31.6	122	74.5	80.5
Giant	54	37	45	137	94	114

Crate and pen sizes recommended for recovery

Use the breed chart opposite as a guide when choosing your dog's crate or pen.

Early Rest and Late Rest

It's usually best to start with a smaller crate or pen (Early Rest), and then move to a larger one after around three weeks (Late Rest). Check with your vet. At each stage, the ideal floor area depends on the size and shape of your dog.

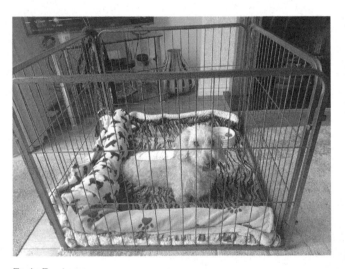

Early Rest pen

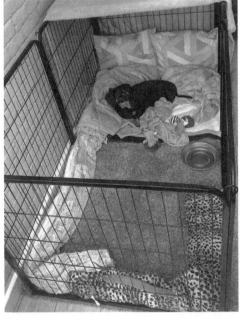

Late Rest pen

→ See Chapter 18 for more information.

Breed chart including recommended sizes of crate and pen

BREED	EARLY REST				LATE REST			
	CRATE SIZE	PEN SHAPE	PEN SIDE LENGTH		CRATE SIZE	PEN SHAPE	PEN SIDE LENGTH	
			CM	INCHES			CM	INCHES
Basset hound	Giant	Square Hexagon	100 to 110 80	40 to 43 32	Avoid crate	Square Octagon	140 to 160 80	55 to 63 32
Beagle	XXL	Square Hexagon Rectangle	80 to 100 80 80 x160	32 to 40 32 32 x 63	Giant	Square Rectangle Octagon	120 to 160 80x160 80	47 x 63 32 x 63 32
Bichon frise	XL	Square	70 to 80	28 to 32	XXL	Rectangle Hexagon	80 x 160 60 to 80	32 x 63 24 to 32
Border collie	XXL * Giant	Square Rectangle	100 to 110 80 x160 *	40 to 43 32 x 63 *	Avoid crate	Square Octagon	140 to 160 80	55 to 63 32
Cavalier King Charles spaniel	XL or XXL	Square	80	32	XXL or giant	Rectangle Hexagon	80 x 160 70 to 80	32 x 63 28 to 32
Chihuahua	L	Square	55	22	XXL	Rectangle Hexagon	55 x 110 50 to 55	22 x 43 20 to 22
Chinese crested dog	XL	Square	70 to 80	28 to 32	XXL	Rectangle Hexagon	80 x 160 60 to 80	32 x 63 24 to 32
Dachshund, miniature	XL	Square	70 to 80	28 to 32	XXL	Rectangle Hexagon	80 x 160 70 to 80	32 x 63 28 to 32
Dachshund, standard	XL or XXL	Square	80 to 100	32 to 40	Avoid crate	Rectangle Hexagon	80 x 160 80	32 x 63 32
French bulldog	XL	Square	70 to 80	28 to 32	XXL	Rectangle Hexagon	80 x 160 70 to 80	32 x 63 28 to 32
Jack Russell terrier	XL	Square	70 to 80	28 to 32	XXL	Rectangle Hexagon	80 x 160 70 to 80	32 x 63 28 to 32
Labrador retriever	Giant	Square Rectangle	110 to 130 80 x 160 *	43 to 51 32 x 63	Avoid crate	Square Rectangle Octagon	160 110 x 220 80	63 43 x 87 32
Lhasa apso	XL	Square	70 to 80	28 to 32	XXL	Rectangle Hexagon	80 x 160 80	32 x 63 32
Maltese	L or XL	Square	70	28	XXL	Rectangle Hexagon	70 x 140 70 to 80	28 x 55 28 to 32
Miniature poodle	XL	Square	80	32	XXL	Rectangle Hexagon	80 x 160 80	32 x 63 32
Miniature schnauzer	XL	Square	80	32	XXL	Rectangle Hexagon	80 x 160 80	32 x 63 32
Nova Scotia duck tolling retriever	Giant	Square Rectangle	100 to 110 80 x 160 *	40 to 43 32 x 63	Avoid crate	Square Octagon	140 to 160 80	55 to 63 32
Pekingese	XL	Square	70 to 80	28 to 32	XXL	Rectangle Hexagon	70 x 140 70	28 x 55 28
Pug	XL	Square	70 to 80	28 to 32	XXL	Rectangle Hexagon	80 x 160 70	32 x 63 28
Shih Tzu	XL	Square	70	28	XXL	Rectangle Hexagon	80 x 160 70	32 x 63 28
Springer spaniel	Giant	Square Rectangle	100 to 110 80 x 160 *	40 to 43 32 x 63	Avoid crate	Square Octagon	140 to 160 80	55 to 63 32
Tibetan spaniel	XL	Square	70 to 80	28 to 32	XLL	Rectangle Hexagon	80 x 160 70	32 x 63 28
Welsh Corgi	XXL* or Giant	Square Rectangle	80* to 100 80 x 160 *	32 to 40 32 x 63	Avoid crate	Square Octagon	120 to 160 80	47 to 63 32

*This space may be too narrow for larger dogs of this breed to turn comfortably.

APPENDIX 5
Posture workouts

TOP TIPS

Posture workouts

✓ Learn the exercises gradually, starting with standing practice (Chapter 58).

✓ Get confident with standing practice before starting to introduce the numbered exercises in Chapter 59. Check first with a physiotherapist if needed.

✓ Add in no more than 2 new exercises per week.

✓ Focus on quality rather than quantity – it's better to do one exercise well than to do several exercises badly.

✓ Watch for signs of tiring (see box 1). Cut the workout short if needed.

Many dogs enjoy the challenge of moving between standing, sitting and sphinx positions, especially if rewarded with a food morsel for each new position. Exercise combinations help train your dog to move between useful postures. For instructions, see:

→ **Chapter 58, 'Standing practice'**

→ **Chapter 59, 'Further posture exercises'**

Once you and your dog are confident with several posture exercises, start to link them into a sequence.

BOX 1: SIGNS OF TIRING

- Knuckling their paws upside-down more often than before

- Becoming less steady on their feet as the exercise continues

- Muscle tremor in the hind legs

- Becoming less cooperative as the exercise continues

If your dog is getting tired, cut the session short.

 TIP: *Work with a helper to turn this into a game. Your dog gets a reward every time they sit, stand, or lie down on command.*

WORKOUT 1: STAND AND SIT

1. Standing practice (Chapter 58) for 10 seconds.
2. Stand to sit (Exercise 3). Sit for 10 seconds.
3. Sit to stand (Exercise 4). Stand for 10 seconds.
4. Stand to sit. Sit for 10 seconds.
5. Lower gently to the floor for a rest.

WORKOUT 2: STAND, SIT AND STANDING EXERCISES

1. Standing practice (Chapter 58) for 10 seconds.
2. Small backward weight shift (Exercise 2).
3. Stand to sit (Exercise 3). Sit for 5 seconds.
4. Sit to stand (Exercise 4). Stand for 10 seconds.
5. Optional – hind paw sequencing (Exercise 1).
6. Stand to sit. Sit for 5 seconds.
7. Lower gently to the floor for a rest.

WORKOUT 3: STAND, SIT AND SITTING EXERCISES

1. Standing practice (Chapter 58) for 10 seconds.
2. Stand to sit (Exercise 3). Sit for 5 seconds.
3. Slow head turn (Exercise 5).
4. Sit to stand (Exercise 4). Stand for 10 seconds.
5. Stand to sit. Sit for 5 seconds.
6. Optional – lift a front paw (Exercise 6).
7. Lower gently to the floor for a rest.

WORKOUT 4: STAND, SIT AND SPHINX

1. Standing practice (Chapter 58) for 10 seconds.
2. Stand to sit (Exercise 3). Sit for 5 seconds.
3. Sit to sphinx (Exercise 7). Sphinx for 10 seconds.
4. Sphinx to sit (Exercise 8). Sit for 5 seconds.
5. Sit to stand (Exercise 4). Stand for 5 seconds.
6. Stand to sit. Sit for 5 seconds.
7. Sit to sphinx.

ADD-INS FOR THE WORKOUTS

Standing parts of the routine can include

✓ hind paw sequencing (Exercise 1)

✓ small backward weight shift (Exercise 2)

✓ slow head turn (Exercise 4)

✓ lifting a front paw (Exercise 6).

Sitting parts of the routine can include

✓ slow head turn (Exercise 4)

✓ lifting a front paw (Exercise 6).

APPENDIX 6
Recovery on a budget

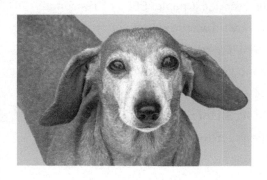

How much does treatment cost?

Treatment for back and neck issues can be very expensive, particularly for dogs that have surgery. Some dogs end up having more than one spinal operation in their lifetime.

Surgical costs

The total hospital fee for a miniature dachshund in the UK, including spinal surgery, an MRI scan just beforehand and in-patient care afterwards, is typically £5,000 to £10,000. This usually includes medication to go home with and one or two routine follow-up appointments. Any problems during follow-up may result in extra costs for further vet consultations and medication.

Cost of non-surgical treatment

Non-surgical treatment generally costs much less than surgery. If you're caring for your dog at home from day one, the main expenses would be vet appointments, prescribed painkillers, and any other medication. Also see below for home care and aftercare costs.

The number of vet check-ups needed depends on your dog's progress. Expect at least two appointments during the first week, and then a minimum of two more during the following month. If your dog has ongoing pain, difficulty peeing, or if their condition is getting worse, more frequent vet check-ups would be needed.

Home care costs

Whether or not you opt for surgery, you'll need the right equipment for home recovery. Essentials include a pen or crate, bedding, non-slip matting if your floors are slippery, a chest harness and lead and, if your dog cannot walk unaided, a hindquarter sling.

Reducing the cost

Let your vet know at the start if you are worried about the cost of treatment. They can then help you choose the most appropriate imaging and treatment options.

Consider non-surgical treatment

Spinal surgery is by far the largest potential cost during IVDD recovery. Consider opting instead for non-surgical treatment. This is a sensible and practical option for many dogs, particularly for those that can walk.

→ For more information, see Chapter 6, 'Should my dog have surgery?'

Avoid spinal X-rays unless they are essential

Spinal X-rays are sometimes offered as a low-cost imaging option for dogs. However, this is often a false economy. If your dog does eventually need an operation, the surgeon would request an MRI or CT scan, even if X-rays have been done. Though cheaper than scans, X-rays still cost several hundred pounds in the UK including the necessary sedative or anaesthetic.

A good reason to have spinal X-rays would be if your vet suspected another condition that would need different treatment, for example a broken back or a disc infection.

→ **For more information, see Chapter 5, 'Diagnostic tests'**

Discuss imaging options with your neurologist

If your dog is to have spinal surgery, they will need imaging just beforehand. It's occasionally possible to reduce costs slightly by doing a CT scan or myelogram instead of an MRI scan. However, these are not appropriate in all cases and are not always available.

Essential treatment at the vet clinic

Remind your vet that you are on a tight budget. They will then know to focus only on essential check-ups and necessary treatment such as prescribed painkillers. Further essential costs depend on how your dog gets on. For example, if your dog cannot pee, they may need extra medication and your vet might need to fit them with a catheter. Consider the following:

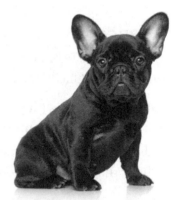

✓ **Focus on good home care.** This helps to prevent common problems during recovery such as skin sores and infections. See sections 8 and 9 for further information.

✓ **Contact your vet for advice straight away if there is a problem**, during standard working hours if possible. If problems occur, it's easier and less expensive to treat them sooner rather than later.

⚠ **BE AWARE:** There's usually an extra fee for seeing a vet out of hours.

Equipment costs

Before buying equipment such as a crate, pen or pushchair, check online. In some cases, it's possible to:

- buy equipment second hand
- loan equipment. A UK charity, 'Dedicated to Dachshunds with IVDD', currently loans pens and other equipment to owners of dachshunds with IVDD.

A key essential expense early in recovery is a pen or large crate. If you cannot loan one or find it second hand in time, you'll need to buy it new. Your dog must be safely confined from the start.

→ **See Appendix 2, 'Shopping lists'**

Avoid unnecessary equipment

Some equipment is popular but unnecessary. For example, as explained in Chapter 69, you don't need a set of stepover poles or a wobble cushion. Your dog could instead walk over a hosepipe or natural safe obstacles during later recovery.

Aftercare costs

The home care advice provided in this book is designed to need minimal equipment and is suitable for dogs recovering on a budget. For general advice, see:

→ **Chapter 10 if they can walk**

→ **Chapters 12-14 if they cannot walk**

Consider extra therapies carefully

Many dogs recover without any extra therapies, just with good home care and prescribed medication.

If you're considering booking acupuncture, hydrotherapy or physiotherapy, mention your limited budget to the therapist from the start. They may be able to space sessions out more widely or to offer a more limited course of treatment.

Avoid paying extra for the following:

- **Machine treatments such as laser.** Dogs recover well without them, and there is little to no evidence that they improve recovery. Though sometimes included as a small part of a physiotherapy programme, it's not worth either buying a machine or visiting a clinic just for a machine treatment.
- **Supplements.** They have not been shown to help dogs with back or neck problems. Instead, ensure that your dog has balanced nutrition by feeding them a diet that is labelled as a 'complete' dog food (Chapter 78).

Insurance

If you have a dachshund, or another breed prone to back or neck problems, good insurance is strongly recommended. Check the small print before choosing.

- Choose a policy with the highest possible level of cover. In the UK, at least £10,000 per year and/or per condition is recommended.
- A lifetime policy is best, as this should cover for recurring problems.
- Check that the policy does not exclude back or neck problems.

Don't wait for your dog to be affected before insuring them. Insurers generally won't cover pre-existing conditions.

If you decide not to take out insurance, consider setting aside regular savings for your dog so that you have money available just in case.

Financial support: further options

Payment plans

It can be worth asking whether your vet clinic can spread costs over a period. However, this is only possible in a few practices.

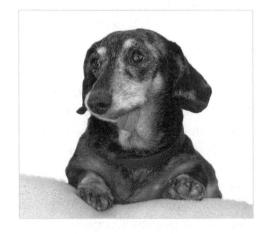

Charitable support

You may be able to get a limited amount of financial support from a charity if you are eligible. However, charities have limited funds so can usually contribute no more than a tiny proportion of the cost of treatment. Check online both for national animal charities and for charitable groups specific to your dog's breed. You can also contact your breed society for advice.

→ See Appendix 12, 'Useful resources'

APPENDIX 7
Other spinal conditions

There are other spinal issues that can have similar effects to IVDD. This table compares some of the more common ones.

SOME SPINAL CONDITIONS

NAME OF CONDITION	TYPICAL ONSET	BREED(S) MOST OFTEN AFFECTED	AGE GROUP MOST OFTEN AFFECTED	USUAL TREATMENT
IVDD: disc extrusion (Hansen Type 1)	sudden	dachshunds, other chondrodystrophic breeds as listed in Chapter 1, box 1	2 years and over	surgery or non-surgical
IVDD: disc protrusion (Hansen Type 2)	gradual	any	over 5 years	surgery or non-surgical
FCE (ischaemic myelopathy or 'spinal stroke')	sudden	any	over 2 years	non-surgical
'Traumatic disc' (ANNPE)	sudden	any	over 2 years	non-surgical
Spinal tumour	sudden or gradual	any	usually older dogs	medical, surgical and/or supportive care depending on exact diagnosis
Discospondylitis	usually gradual	usually larger breeds	usually older dogs	antibiotics and supportive care
Degenerative myelopathy	gradual	German shepherd dog, poodle, boxer, Pembroke Welsh corgi. Can affect any breed	over 8 years	non-surgical – supportive home care
'Pug myelopathy' constrictive myelopathy	gradual	pugs	older adults: average age of onset 7 years	non-surgical – supportive home care; surgery is sometimes also considered

Traumatic disc and FCE

Two conditions can look particularly like sudden-onset IVDD:

1. **Traumatic disc.** This is also called ANNPE which stands for acute non-compressive nucleus pulposus extrusion. It involves a spinal disc exploding suddenly, bruising the spinal cord.
2. **Fibrocartilaginous embolism (FCE).** This is also sometimes called ischaemic myelopathy, and you may also hear it casually referred to as a 'spinal stroke'. FCE is caused by part of the spinal cord losing its blood supply, for example due to a clot in a blood vessel.

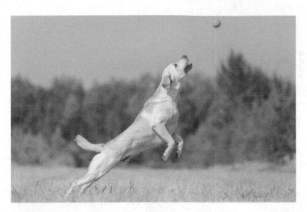

Figure 1: Traumatic disc and FCE tend to happen during or just after a bout of vigorous exercise.

BOX 2: HOME CARE FOR DOGS WITH FCE OR TRAUMATIC DISC

How best to look after your dog depends on how badly they are affected:

→ **If they can walk, see Chapter 10**
→ **If they cannot walk, see Chapters 12-14**

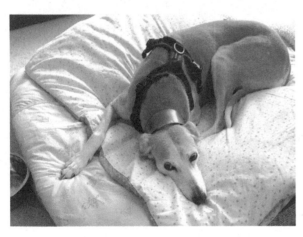

Figure 2: During recovery from FCE or traumatic disc, a comfortable floor bed and non-slip matting are essential.

Both traumatic disc and FCE can cause the dog to be unsteady on their feet, or to collapse with weak or paralysed legs. Many dogs yelp just as the problem first starts, and they may have a painful back or neck when first assessed by the vet. However, any pain resolves within the first day or so in most cases.

Unlike IVDD, these conditions are not inherited, and any breed can be affected. They tend to start suddenly, often while the dog is running around.

Diagnosis

A vet cannot know for sure whether the dog has traumatic disc or FCE, but the presentation and history may give them a very strong suspicion. An MRI scan can usually confirm the diagnosis if needed.

Treatment of FCE and traumatic disc

There is no operation to help these dogs. Instead, they need supportive care that is very similar to non-surgical treatment for IVDD. If your dog has had either FCE or a traumatic disc, set them up in a recovery crate, pen or room (Section 4). Keep them on the lead when outdoors, and use a sling if needed. They may also need help with toileting, as for dogs with IVDD (Section 8).

The good news is that dogs with FCE or traumatic disc are unlikely to get worse. Despite this, it's important to restrict their activity during recovery:

- These dogs are very unsteady on their feet. They are prone to injuring other parts of themselves if allowed to rush about, or if they slip on slick flooring or rest unsupervised on a sofa.

- Dogs soon learn to drag themselves about if allowed to roam free. This can make it more difficult for them to learn to walk properly.

Will my dog recover from FCE or traumatic disc?

After an episode of either condition, around 7 out of 10 dogs do learn to walk again[1]. However, those that are paralysed and have lost pain sensation in their legs have a much lower chance of recovery.

After either a traumatic disc or FCE, around three out of four dogs that learn to walk again are left slightly unsteady on their feet in the long term[2]. A few are also left with imperfect bladder or bowel control.

Many dogs start to improve within the first few days of an FCE or traumatic disc. They may even start walking again as early as one week after the injury. However, recovery times vary, with a few dogs taking more than two months to start walking again. Those that are worst affected tend to take the longest to recover.

1. De Risio et al 2007, 2. Fenn et al 2016

Disc protrusion (Hansen type 2 IVDD)

What do these dogs look like?

Disc protrusion is a type of IVDD mainly seen in older dogs (see Chapter 1). Affected dogs may be less playful than they used to be, and perhaps reluctant to go out for their usual walks. Signs tend to start gradually, though sudden flare-ups are also possible. Some dogs have several discs affected and, being older, they may also have stiff or unstable joints.

Imaging

X-rays can be used to check for other problems such as infection in the discs or osteoarthritis (degeneration of limb joints due to wear and tear). A disc protrusion itself does not show up on X-rays, though your vet might see new bone growth called 'spondylosis' around an affected part of their spine. If your vet needs to confirm the cause of the problem, they could refer your dog for an MRI or CT scan.

> **BOX 3: SIGNS OF DISC PROTRUSION**
>
> - Pain
> - Weak legs: difficulty standing for long, slow to get up off the floor, difficulty jumping or using stairs
> - Odd gait:
>   - you may hear claws dragging as your dog walks, and the claws may get scuffed.
>   - difficulty walking on slick floors
> - Difficulty standing still to pee or poo
> - Muscle wasting, especially over the hind legs

Treatment

> **TOP TIPS**
>
> ### Caring for a dog with disc protrusion
>
> - ✓ **See your vet.** They can assess your dog, prescribe painkillers, and adjust doses as needed.
> - ✓ **Indoor lifestyle changes (chapter 73).** Avoid slick floors, stairs, steps and jumping. Provide good floor beds, and close doors so your dog doesn't rush through the home.
> - ✓ **Outdoor lifestyle changes (chapter 74).** Shorten your dog's walks so they come home no stiffer than they left the house. Take them outdoors for no more than 5 minutes at a time if they are in a very bad way. Avoid all ball games. Use a harness and lead, and encourage your dog to walk slowly.
>
> Routine 6 'Walkers aftercare' is suitable for many dogs with a disc protrusion (see Appendix 1). Each dog has different needs, so check first with your vet
>
> Expect gradual improvement. After putting all the above changes into place, your dog should start to feel at least a little better within the first week, and there should be clear improvement within three weeks. If your dog does not seem to be improving, or if they are getting worse, discuss this with your vet. They may need to adjust painkiller doses or to refer your dog to a neurologist.

Dogs with a disc protrusion are usually cared for non-surgically. In addition to the painkillers and lifestyle changes, a spinal operation is sometimes helpful. However, surgical success rates vary, and are generally lower than for a disc extrusion. If you opt for referral, discuss your own dog's chances of recovery and expected recovery time with the neurologist.

For a general guide to caring for your dog at home after spinal surgery:

→ **See Chapter 10 if your dog can walk after their operation**

→ **See Chapters 12-14 if your dog cannot walk after their operation**

APPENDIX 8
Reducing the risk of IVDD

SUMMARY

✓ Choose a puppy carefully.

✓ Don't neuter them until they are fully grown.

✓ Keep your dog at an ideal weight.

✓ Help your dog stick to a sensible, moderate lifestyle (see box 6).

✓ Be prepared for problems if your breed is prone to IVDD. The condition is not entirely preventable.

Choosing a dog with less risk of IVDD

Some breeds such as dachshunds and French bulldogs are born with a high risk of getting back and neck issues. Crossbreeds of these dogs can also be affected. If you are reading this book then this advice may come too late, but to avoid IVDD it's best to choose a breed that is less prone to problems.

→ **For a list of at-risk breeds, see Chapter 1, 'What is IVDD'.**

Choosing a puppy of an at-risk breed

There is no reliable way to prevent or avoid IVDD. However, it's worth checking the following before buying:

❧ Ask the breeder whether close relatives of the pup's parents have had back or neck problems. IVDD tends to run in families.

❧ For dachshunds in the UK, Scandinavia, Australia, New Zealand and South Africa, ask the breeder whether the parents have had spinal X-rays as part of the IVDD screening programme (see box 4).

❧ For French bulldogs in the UK and Australia, ask the breeder whether the parents have had spinal X-rays to check for 'congenital vertebral malformations' which may be passed on to pups. These are abnormally shaped spinal bones that sometimes lead to problems including IVDD.

❧ For other breeds at risk of IVDD, ask your local or national kennel club. They can advise on whether the DNA test for IVDD is useful in your breed (see box 5).

BOX 4: IVDD X-RAY SCREENING PROGRAMME FOR DACHSHUND BREEDERS

In UK and Scandinavia, the X-ray screening programme helps to produce dachshund puppies that are less prone to IVDD. Dogs are X-rayed at 2 to 4 years old to check for abnormal calcified discs in their spine. Most dachshunds have at least one calcified disc, but some have more than others.

Dogs with high numbers of calcified discs should not be used for breeding. Not only are these dogs more likely to get back trouble themselves, but they are more likely to pass it on to future generations.

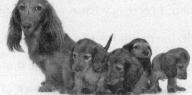

Avoid early neutering

A study looking at around two thousand dachshunds[1] found that males and females neutered before 12 months old were more likely to go on to get back or neck disease. This may also be true for other breeds, as changing hormone levels affect the degeneration of discs in the spine.

Lifestyle to reduce risk of back problems

✓ Aim for moderate daily activities (see box 6) to reduce wear and tear on the joints, muscles and spine. This is not guaranteed to prevent IVDD, but is sensible advice for all dogs.

✓ Keep your dog at a healthy body weight (see Chapter 79, 'Is my dog overweight?'). Studies suggest that overweight dogs are more likely to have an episode of IVDD.

✓ Avoid repetitive, high impact sports.

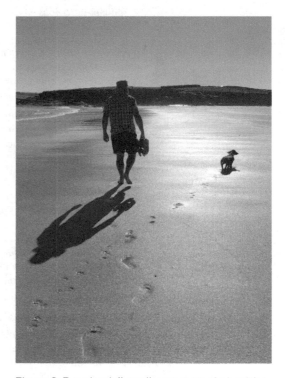

Figure 3: Regular daily walks are part of a healthy lifestyle.

1. Dorn & Seath 2018

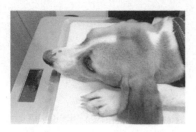

Figure 4: Weigh your dog regularly.

Weight management

Keeping your dog at an ideal weight will reduce the risk of IVDD-related problems. For dachshunds, use the body condition score chart below to check whether they are under or overweight.

→ **See Chapter 79 for more information.**

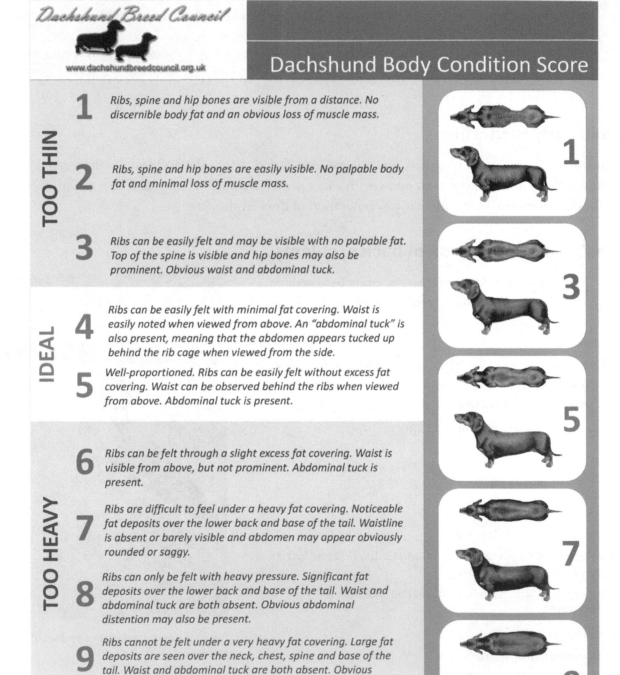

Dachshund Breed Council
www.dachshundbreedcouncil.org.uk

Dachshund Body Condition Score

TOO THIN

1 Ribs, spine and hip bones are visible from a distance. No discernible body fat and an obvious loss of muscle mass.

2 Ribs, spine and hip bones are easily visible. No palpable body fat and minimal loss of muscle mass.

3 Ribs can be easily felt and may be visible with no palpable fat. Top of the spine is visible and hip bones may also be prominent. Obvious waist and abdominal tuck.

IDEAL

4 Ribs can be easily felt with minimal fat covering. Waist is easily noted when viewed from above. An "abdominal tuck" is also present, meaning that the abdomen appears tucked up behind the rib cage when viewed from the side.

5 Well-proportioned. Ribs can be easily felt without excess fat covering. Waist can be observed behind the ribs when viewed from above. Abdominal tuck is present.

TOO HEAVY

6 Ribs can be felt through a slight excess fat covering. Waist is visible from above, but not prominent. Abdominal tuck is present.

7 Ribs are difficult to feel under a heavy fat covering. Noticeable fat deposits over the lower back and base of the tail. Waistline is absent or barely visible and abdomen may appear obviously rounded or saggy.

8 Ribs can only be felt with heavy pressure. Significant fat deposits over the lower back and base of the tail. Waist and abdominal tuck are both absent. Obvious abdominal distention may also be present.

9 Ribs cannot be felt under a very heavy fat covering. Large fat deposits are seen over the neck, chest, spine and base of the tail. Waist and abdominal tuck are both absent. Obvious abdominal distention.

For more information and tips on caring for your Dachshund, visit:
www.dachshundbreedcouncil.org.uk and www.dachshundhealth.org.uk
© 2020 Dachshund Health UK (Registered Charity 1177400)
Body condition images by Hannah James.

Safer sports

If your dog is keen to do something sporty, consider Canine Hoopers. This has been developed as a low-impact version of dog agility. It involves wide turns, tunnels, and hoops instead of jumps.

Back braces

Back braces wrap around the dog's body and are sometimes sold for dogs with IVDD to help support the spine. However, braces have not been shown to prevent recurrence of back problems or to improve recovery.

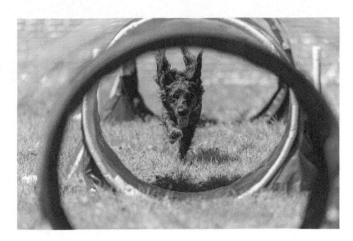

Figure 5: Canine Hoopers.

If you decide to try your dog with a back brace, be cautious and continue to restrict their activity. Fabric braces are slightly flexible and don't completely stabilise the dog's back. And they don't offer any neck support. This could leave your dog prone to further problems, especially if they leap and jump about.

Being prepared for back problems

You can avoid much of the worry and heartbreak caused by back or neck problems by being prepared.

Financial planning

If you have a dachshund, or another breed prone to IVDD, set aside funds just in case. This can make all the difference between being able to care for your dog and having to make a difficult decision. It's well worth arranging good insurance while your dog is still healthy.

→ See Appendix 6, 'Recovery on a budget'.

Being prepared

Have some basic first aid equipment at home:

* a fixed length dog lead
* a chest harness that fits your dog
* something that could be used as a sling in an emergency
* non-slip mats if your floors are slippery
* a pen or large crate. Many types fold flat for storage.

Recovery is easier if your dog:

✓ is accustomed to being in a crate or pen for short periods now and again

✓ has been trained not to jump on and off the furniture, or can use a ramp or sofa steps

✓ does not expect to use stairs regularly.

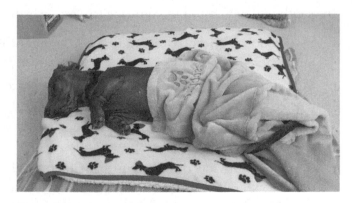

Figure 6: Recovery is easier if your dog is used to sleeping at floor level downstairs.

APPENDIX 9
Thinking about euthanasia

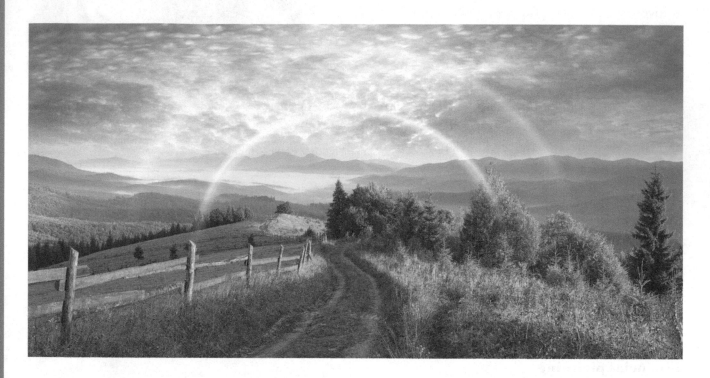

Is it time to make the decision?

If your dog is badly affected by IVDD, and if there is no appropriate, realistic or effective treatment available, then you may unfortunately have to consider the last resort option of euthanasia – having them put to sleep. Sometimes this is the only kind choice to make on behalf of our pets, to save them from further pain.

Don't be rushed into this important decision. You can ask your vet to let you think about it, at least overnight. In many cases, it's sensible to take the dog home for a day or so on prescribed painkillers while you decide what to do next. If you have spoken to your vet and feel the need to talk things through with someone else at this point, consider contacting an IVDD support group (see Appendix 12).

In deciding whether to put your dog to sleep, weigh up the different issues:

- If your dog is given treatment that you can afford, do they have any chance of returning to a reasonable quality of life?

- Will you be able to care for your dog during recovery, and if not, are there people who can be trusted to help you? Basic care and nursing skills can be learned and will soon become routine. However, some owners cannot care for a recovering dog, for example due to their own illness, long working hours or caring responsibilities.

- If vets are convinced that your dog will not walk again, could they go on to live a happy life on wheels? Note that some dogs that cannot walk will also have long term incontinence problems. Consider if this is manageable given both your lifestyle and your dog's personality.

Euthanasia: a few notes on practicalities

When booking a final appointment, let the practice know that you need to have your dog put to sleep. Veterinary staff will be sympathetic and try their best to allocate enough time and ensure that everyone is prepared. Some practices might even be able to arrange a home visit. Another option could be to arrange a home visit from a mobile veterinary euthanasia service if one covers your area.

If you take your dog to the clinic, bring their bed or a familiar blanket or towel for them to rest on. There's usually the option to stay in the room with the dog during euthanasia so that you can say goodbye. Just let your vet know if you prefer to slip out at any stage or indeed if you'd rather not be present at all.

Think about cremation and burial options in advance if you can. Ask the receptionist or practice manager what is available. Most practices offer cremation. For an extra fee, it may be possible to have ashes returned to you either in a tube for scattering or in an urn. Other options may include home burial if you have a suitable garden, or burial in a pet cemetery.

Afterwards

Each owner experiences the pain of losing their dog differently. Some are overwhelmed by grief, while others feel more shocked or angry at what has happened. It's also normal to be left feeling lonely and 'empty', or unable to think straight for a while. Be patient with yourself. It takes a different length of time for everyone, but this sad time will eventually pass.

You may find it helpful to:

* **Look after yourself** – eat properly, stay hydrated, and continue to get outdoors.
* **Spend time with people** who care about you.
* **Commemorate your dog** in some way – for example, plant a tree in their memory, scatter their ashes somewhere meaningful to you, or fill a box with items connected to them.
* **If you have other pets**, try to continue their routines as normal.
* **Connect with others** on IVDD or pet loss support groups. Other dog owners will understand something of what you are going through.
* **Call a pet loss hotline** if you need to talk to someone aside from your friends and family (Appendix 12).
* **Look back through photos and other memories** of your dog once you feel ready. It is okay to cry if you find yourself doing so. You might also eventually smile or laugh at the happier memories.

APPENDIX 10
Clinical studies

Treatments should be tested in studies to find out whether they work. Significant improvement in a large percentage of patients in good quality studies suggests that the treatment works. Good studies involve the following:

- **Control group.** Treated dogs should be compared with those that didn't get treatment. For example, dogs having physiotherapy after surgery could be compared with those having surgery but no physiotherapy.

- **Placebo group.** This is a control group that is given a pretend treatment. Studies have shown that there is a placebo effect in dogs, which means that those given a pretend treatment appear to improve[1,2].

  For example, some dogs in a study are given a tablet as a treatment. Others might instead be given a sugar pill as a placebo. The sugar pill is not expected to affect their recovery. Researchers then see whether the dogs given the treatment recover faster than those given the sugar pill.

> **A placebo is a 'pretend' treatment that looks just like the real one. It's used in some studies to help check whether a treatment is effective.**

To test a supplement, the effect of the true supplement should be compared with a placebo, an identical-looking tablet that contains no active ingredient. To investigate laser, therapy with a true laser can be compared with sham laser using a machine that looks identical but does not produce a laser beam.

- **Blind studies.** Studies should be 'blinded'. This means that people involved are not told whether the dog is getting the real or pretend (placebo) treatment until the study is complete. This should include those assessing the dog's outcome, owners giving the treatment, and clinicians handing the treatment to the owner.

- **A large number of dogs.** Successful treatment of a few dogs may just be down to chance. Improvement in many dogs is more likely to suggest that the treatment works.

- **Standardised patients.** All the dogs in the study should have the same condition and be at the same stage of recovery. If studies have not been done on dogs, we can look at studies on humans or other animals.

- **Standardised treatment.** All the dogs in the treatment group should get the same dose of a supplement, or the same type of therapy.

- **Randomization.** Once selected for the study, dogs should be put into the treatment and control groups at random.

- **No conflict of interest.** Beware of studies that are performed or funded by companies that sell a supplement or treatment. These can be biased.

- **Repeatable results.** The true effect of the treatment remains uncertain if one study suggests that a treatment works, while another suggests that it doesn't.

1. Conzemius et al 2012, 2. Muñana et al 2010

APPENDIX 11
References

Chapter 83: Physiotherapy

1. Li, Z., Yao, F., Cheng, L., Cheng, W., Qi, L., Yu, S., Zhang L., Zha X., & Jing, J. (2019). Low frequency pulsed electromagnetic field promotes the recovery of neurological function after spinal cord injury in rats. *Journal of Orthopaedic Research*, 37(2), 449-456.

2. Alvarez, L. X., McCue, J., Lam, N. K., Askin, G., & Fox, P. R. (2019). Effect of targeted pulsed electromagnetic field therapy on canine postoperative hemilaminectomy: a double-blind, randomized, placebo-controlled clinical trial. *Journal of the American Animal Hospital Association*, 55(2), 83-91.

3. Zidan, N., Fenn, J., Griffith, E., Early, P. J., Mariani, C. L., Munana, K. R., Guevar J., & Olby, N. J. (2018). The effect of electromagnetic fields on post-operative pain and locomotor recovery in dogs with acute, severe thoracolumbar intervertebral disc extrusion: a randomized placebo-controlled, prospective clinical trial. *Journal of neurotrauma*, 35(15), 1726-1736.

4. Chen, L., Xing, F., Liu, G., Gong, M., Li, L., Chen, R., & Xiang, Z. (2019). Effects of pulsed electromagnetic field therapy on pain, stiffness and physical function in patients with knee osteoarthritis: a systematic review and meta-analysis of randomized controlled trials. *Journal of rehabilitation medicine*, 51(11), 821-827.

5. Piao, D., Sypniewski, L. A., Dugat, D., Bailey, C., Burba, D. J., & De Taboada, L. (2019). Transcutaneous transmission of photobiomodulation light to the spinal canal of dog as measured from cadaver dogs using a multi-channel intra-spinal probe. *Lasers in medical science*, 34(8), 1645-1654.

6. Stephens, B., Baltzer W., Harrington, P. (2011). Internal Dosimetry: Combining Simulation with Phantom and Ex Vivo Measurement

7. Tomazoni, S. S., Almeida, M. O., Bjordal, J. M., Stausholm, M. B., Machado, C. D. S. M., Leal-Junior, E. C. P., & Costa, L. O. P. (2020). Photobiomodulation therapy does not decrease pain and disability in people with non-specific low back pain: a systematic review. *Journal of Physiotherapy*, 66(3), 155-165.

8. Kadhim-Saleh, A., Maganti, H., Ghert, M., Singh, S., & Farrokhyar, F. (2013). Is low-level laser therapy in relieving neck pain effective? Systematic review and meta-analysis. *Rheumatology international*, 33(10), 2493-2501.

Chapter 85: Nutritional supplements

1. Stuber, K., Sajko, S., & Kristmanson, K. (2011). Efficacy of glucosamine, chondroitin, and methylsulfonylmethane for spinal degenerative joint disease and degenerative disc disease: a systematic review. *The Journal of the Canadian Chiropractic Association*, 55(1), 47.

2. Philippi, A. F., Leffler, C. T., Leffler, S. G., Mosure, J. C., & Kim, P. D. (1999). Glucosamine, chondroitin, and manganese ascorbate for degenerative joint disease of the knee or low back: a randomized, double-blind, placebo-controlled pilot study. *Military medicine*, 164(2), 85-91.

3. Anand, P., Kunnumakkara, A. B., Newman, R. A., & Aggarwal, B. B. (2007). Bioavailability of curcumin: problems and promises. Molecular pharmaceutics, 4(6), 807-818.

4. Innes, J. F., Fuller, C. J., Grover, E. R., Kelly, A. L., & Burn, J. F. (2003). Randomised, double-blind, placebo controlled parallel group study of P54FP for the treatment of dogs with osteoarthritis. *Veterinary Record*, 152(15), 457-460.

Appendix 3: Clinical grade chart

1. Aikawa, T., Fujita, H., Kanazono, S., Shibata, M., & Yoshigae, Y. (2012). Long-term neurologic outcome of hemilaminectomy and disk fenestration for treatment of dogs with thoracolumbar intervertebral disk herniation: 831 cases (2000–2007). *Journal of the American Veterinary Medical Association*, 241(12), 1617-1626.

2. Davies, J. V., & Sharp, N. J. H. (1983). A comparison of conservative treatment and

fenestration for thoracolumbar intervertebral disc disease in the dog. *Journal of Small Animal Practice*, 24(12), 721-729.

3. Hayashi, A. M., Matera, J. M., & de Campos Fonseca, A. C. B. (2007). Evaluation of electroacupuncture treatment for thoracolumbar intervertebral disk disease in dogs. *Journal of the American Veterinary Medical Association*, 231(6), 913-918.

4. Ingram, E. A., Kale, D. C., & Balfour, R. J. (2013). Hemilaminectomy for thoracolumbar Hansen Type I intervertebral disk disease in ambulatory dogs with or without neurologic deficits: 39 cases (2008–2010). *Veterinary Surgery*, 42(8), 924-931.

5. Jeong, I. S., Rahman, M. M., Kim, H., Lee, G. J., Seo, B. S., Choi, G. C., Kim S., & Kim, N. (2018). Prognostic value with intervertebral herniation disk disease in dogs. *Journal of Advanced Veterinary and Animal Research*, 5(2), 240-246.

6. Kazakos, G., Polizopoulou, Z. S., Patsikas, M. N., Tsimopoulos, G., Roubies, N., & Dessiris, A. (2005). Duration and severity of clinical signs as prognostic indicators in 30 dogs with thoracolumbar disk disease after surgical decompression. *Transboundary and Emerging Diseases*, 52(3), 147-152.

7. Langerhuus, L., & Miles, J. (2017). Proportion recovery and times to ambulation for non-ambulatory dogs with thoracolumbar disc extrusions treated with hemilaminectomy or conservative treatment: A systematic review and meta-analysis of case-series studies. *The Veterinary Journal*, 220, 7-16.

8. Levine, J. M., Levine, G. J., Johnson, S. I., Kerwin, S. C., Hettlich, B. F., & Fosgate, G. T. (2007). Evaluation of the success of medical management for presumptive thoracolumbar intervertebral disk herniation in dogs. *Veterinary surgery*, 36(5), 482-491.

9. Mann, F. A., Wagner-Mann, C. C., Dunphy, E. D., Ruben, D. S., Rochat, M. C., & Bartels, K. E. (2007). Recurrence rate of presumed thoracolumbar intervertebral disc disease in ambulatory dogs with spinal hyperpathia treated with anti-inflammatory drugs: 78 cases (1997–2000). *Journal of Veterinary Emergency and Critical Care*, 17(1), 53-60.

10. Nečas, A. (1999). Clinical aspects of surgical treatment of thoracolumbar disc disease in dogs. A retrospective study of 300 cases. *Acta Veterinaria Brno*, 68(2), 121-130.

11. Sukhiani, H. R., Parent, J. M., Atilola, M. A., & Holmberg, D. L. (1996). Intervertebral disk disease in dogs with signs of back pain alone: 25 cases (1986-1993). *Journal of the American Veterinary Medical Association*, 209(7), 1275-1279.

12. Sedlacek, J., Rychel, J., Giuffrida, M., & Wright, B. (2022). Nonsurgical Rehabilitation in Dachshunds With T3-L3 Myelopathy: Prognosis and Rates of Recurrence. *Frontiers in Veterinary Science*, 955.

Appendix 7: Other conditions

1. De Risio, L. D., Adams, V., Dennis, R., McConnell, F., & Platt, S. (2007). Magnetic resonance imaging findings and clinical associations in 52 dogs with suspected ischemic myclopathy. *Journal of veterinary internal medicine*, 21(6), 1290-1298.

2. Fenn, J., Drees, R., Volk, H. A., & De Decker, S. (2016). Comparison of clinical signs and outcomes between dogs with presumptive ischemic myelopathy and dogs with acute noncompressive nucleus pulposus extrusion. *Journal of the American Veterinary Medical Association*, 249(7), 767-775.

Appendix 8: Reducing the risk of IVDD

1. Dorn, M., & Seath, I. J. (2018). Neuter status as a risk factor for canine intervertebral disc herniation (IVDH) in dachshunds: a retrospective cohort study. *Canine genetics and epidemiology*, 5(1), 1-14.

Appendix 10: Clinical studies

1. Conzemius, M. G., & Evans, R. B. (2012). Caregiver placebo effect for dogs with lameness from osteoarthritis. *Journal of the American Veterinary Medical Association*, 241(10), 1314-1319.

2. Muñana, K. R., Zhang, D., & Patterson, E. E. (2010). Placebo effect in canine epilepsy trials. *Journal of veterinary internal medicine*, 24(1), 166-170.

APPENDIX 12
Useful resources

Registers of certified clinicians (UK)

Acupuncture

- **ABVA** Association of British Veterinary Acupuncturists: abva.co.uk
- **IVAS** International Veterinary Acupuncture Society: ivas.org

Behaviour Counsellors

- **ABTC** Animal Behaviour and Training Council: abtc.org.uk
- **APBC** Association of Pet Behaviour Counsellors: apbc.org.uk
- **ASAB** Association for the Study of Animal Behaviour: asab.org/ccab
- **FABC** Fellowship of Animal Behaviour Clinicians: fabclinicians.org
- **IAABC** International Association of Animal Behavior Consultants: m.iaabc.org

Hydrotherapists

- **CHA** Canine Hydrotherapy Association: canine-hydrotherapy.org
- **NARCH** National Association of Registered Canine Hydrotherapists: narch.org.uk/Home/Index

Physiotherapists

- **ACPAT** Association of Chartered Physiotherapists in Animal Therapy: acpat.org
- **IRVAP** Institute of Registered Veterinary and Animal Physiotherapists: irvap.org.uk
- **RAMP** Register of Animal Musculoskeletal Practitioners: rampregister.org

Equipment

- **Archie's Workshop** (dog ramps and pet steps): ArchiesWorkshop.com
- **Dedicated to Dachshunds with IVDD** (for UK dachshund owners only – a charity offering equipment loans and basic advice): dedicatedtodachshunds.co.uk
- **Eddie's Wheels** (bespoke wheels for dogs that cannot walk): EddiesWheels.com
- **Help 'Em Up harness** available from:
  - **Orthopets Europe:** orthopets.co.uk/mobility-solutions/help-emup
  - **Paw Prosper:** helpemup.com
- **Perfect fit harness:** perfect-fit-dog-harness.com

Online information

- **Dachshund Health UK.** Information on this website includes details of the X-ray breeding scheme and a list of referral practices recommended by dachshund owners: dachshund-ivdd.uk

- **The Rehab Vet** (the author's website and online resource): therehabvet.com

Online support groups

- **Dachshund IVDD UK:** facebook.com/groups/VITALDachshundIVDD

- **Dedicated to Dachshunds:** facebook.com/Dedicatedtodachshunds

- **Dodgerslist – Disc Disease – IVDD Education and Support:** facebook.com/Dodgerslist

- **French bulldog IVDD support:** facebook.com/groups/178483559398659

- **IVDD and Other Back Disorders in Dogs:** facebook.com/groups/408512465849039

Charities (UK)

- **Blue cross:** bluecross.org.uk/veterinary

- **Dogs trust:** moretodogstrust.org.uk

- **PDSA:** pdsa.org.uk

- **RSPCA:** rspca.org.uk

Pet loss helplines

- **Pet Bereavement Support Service** (UK) 0800 096 6606

- **ASPCA** Pet Loss helpline (US) 877-474-3310

- **Chance's Spot** – Pet loss and grief support – includes a webpage with further helplines: chancesspot.org/hotlines.php

Education

- **K9HS Courses,** recommended for canine therapists to progress and advance their clinical skills: k9hscourses.com

Low impact canine sport

- **Canine Hoopers UK:** caninehoopersuk.co.uk

- **Canine Hoopers World:** caninehoopersworld.com

GLOSSARY

Ambulatory Able to walk without help or support.

Analgesics Painkillers.

Ataxia Loss of coordination. In dogs with IVDD, this may involve paws placed upside down, legs crossing while walking, or staggering like a drunk person.

Cervical Involving the neck.

Chondrodystrophy An inherited condition that interferes with the body's normal cartilage development. Chondrodystrophic breeds tend to have short legs and are more prone to IVDD.

Congenital Vertebral Malformation (CVM) A vertebra that has an unusual shape from birth. For example, it might have a piece missing. CVMs may show up on X-ray in dogs that are otherwise healthy. They are often seen in French bulldogs and pugs. Dogs with CVMs are more likely to get other spinal conditions such as IVDD.

CT (computerised tomography) A type of scan that produces detailed images of the inside of the body. It uses a computer to combine the results of X-rays taken from many different angles.

Disc herniation. A disc that has bulged or ruptured is said to have 'herniated'. This could either be an extrusion (Hansen type 1 herniation) or a protrusion (Hansen type 2 herniation). See Chapter 1.

Disc prolapse = disc herniation.

Discs (disks in US) Pad-like structures between adjacent vertebrae (bones in the spine). They cushion the vertebrae as the dog moves.

Fenestration A type of spinal surgery that could reduce the risk of disc extrusion recurring.

Hemilaminectomy A type of spinal surgery often used in the mid-back region. It reduces pressure on the spinal cord.

Heritable Refers to any condition that can be passed from parents to offspring.

Inflammation The body's natural response to injury or infection. The affected area becomes swollen, painful and reddened and may feel warmer than usual.

Ischaemic (ischemic) myelopathy Damage to the spinal cord caused by a reduced blood supply.

IVDD (intervertebral disc disease) A condition affecting the back or neck. IVDD includes disc degeneration, any type of disc herniation that this may cause, and the pain and other problems caused by this. See Chapter 1.

IVDE (intervertebral disc extrusion) A type of IVDD in which the centre of a degenerated disc pushes out through a split in the outer layer, pressing against the spinal cord and damaging it.

IVDH (intervertebral disc herniation) Another term for disc herniation.

Lumbar Involving the lower back.

Lumbosacral Involving the region between the lumbar spine (lower back) and the sacrum (the section of the spine in the pelvic area).

Meninges Sheets of tissue (membranes) around the spinal cord and brain.

Motor control A dog's control of their own deliberate movements.

MRI (magnetic resonance imaging) A type of scan that produces detailed images of the inside of the body. It uses a strong magnetic field and radio waves.

Myelography A specialised X-ray procedure in which dye is injected into the spinal canal so that the spinal cord becomes visible.

Myelomalacia Softening of the spinal cord (see Appendix 3).

Neural Relating to nerve cells or to the nervous system.

Neurologist A vet with special expertise in treating conditions involving the spine, brain and nerves.

Non-ambulatory Unable to walk without support.

NSAIDs (Non-steroidal anti-inflammatory drugs) A type of painkiller that reduces inflammation.

Paralysis Inability to make any deliberate muscle movements. One or more legs may be affected.

Paraparesis Muscle weakness (paresis) that only involves the hind legs.

Paresis Muscle weakness caused by nerve damage. Partial paralysis affecting one or more legs.

Patellar luxation 'Slipping kneecap'. A condition often seen in small breeds including mini dachshunds. It tends to cause hopping or missed steps. Signs usually start in puppies or young adults. Patellar luxation may worsen after a bout of IVDD because of changes in muscle tone.

Proprioception A dog's awareness of where their body is and of how it is moving.

Radiography Imaging of the inside of the body using X-rays.

Reflex movement Automatic movement in response to a stimulus such as having a toe pinched. Reflex movement is not conscious or deliberate and is controlled by nerve pathways that do not involve the brain.

Sacral nerve stimulator Currently with very limited availability, this new technique helps some dogs that have failed to regain bladder control. A specialist operates on the dog, implanting a small device close to the bladder's nerve-supply. Back home, the owner can then prompt the dog to urinate using a hand-held remote control.

Spinal arachnoid diverticulum (SAD) A pocket of fluid that builds up above the spinal cord and presses on it. Most often seen in French bulldogs and pugs.

Spinal cord A long cord of nerve cells running through the spine. The spinal cord is the main pathway for information travelling between the brain and the rest of the body.

Spine The spine is made up of bones called vertebrae. The spine protects and supports the spinal cord in the dog's neck and back.

Spondylosis New bone growth around the spine, often seen on X-rays of older dogs.

Thoracic Involving the region of the spine at the level of the chest.

Thoracolumbar Involving the regions of the spine at the level of the chest and lower back.

Ventral slot procedure A type of spinal surgery often used in the neck. It reduces pressure on the spinal cord.

Vertebrae The bones making up the spine.

Voluntary movement Purposeful, deliberate movement.

Index

Made in the USA
Coppell, TX
26 November 2023